Cardiology Research and Clinical Developments

nova
Medicine & Health
New York

Cardiology Research and Clinical Developments

Pericarditis: From Diagnosis to Treatment
Nicholas Clément (Editor)
2022. ISBN: 978-1-68507-764-8 (Softcover)
2022. ISBN: 978-1-68507-960-4 (eBook)

Heart Transplantation: Indications, Postoperative Management and Long-Term Outcomes
Elian Facundo Giordanino, MD (Editor)
2022. ISBN: 978-1-68507-759-4 (Hardcover)
2022. ISBN: 978-1-68507-941-3 (eBook)

Perspectives in Aortic Valve Disease: Clinical and Morphological Characteristics, Diagnosis and Treatments
Giovanni Concistrè (Editor)
2020. ISBN: 978-1-53618-769-4 (Hardcover)
2020. ISBN: 978-1-53618-848-6 (eBook)

The Interventional Cardiology World: User's Manual of the Cath. Lab. for Students and Apprentices
Dario Buccheri, MD (Editor)
Bernardo Cortese (Editor)
Alessio La Manna, MD (Editor)
2020. ISBN: 978-1-53618-249-1 (Hardcover)
2020. ISBN: 978-1-53618-675-8 (eBook)

More information about this series can be found at
https://novapublishers.com/product-category/series/cardiology-research-and-clinical-developments/

Irena Mitevska
Sonja Salinger
Marijan Bosevski
Elizabeta Srbinovska
and Slobodan Obradovic
Editors

Pulmonary Embolism

Contemporary Diagnosis, Risk Stratification and Management

Medicine & Health
New York

Library of Congress Cataloging-in-Publication Data

Names: Mitevska, Irena, editor. | Salinger, Sonja, editor. | Bosevski, Marijan, editor. | Srbinovska, Elizabeta, editor. | Obradovic, Slobodan, editor.
Title: Pulmonary embolism: contemporary diagnosis, risk stratification and management / Irena Mitevska, MD, PhD, editor, Associate Professor, Vice President of the National Society of Cardiology of North Macedonia, Intensive Care Unit, University Cardiological Clinic, Skopje, North Macedonia, Sonja Salinger, editor, Associate Professor of Cardiology, Cardiology Clinic, Clinical Center of Nis, Serbia.
Description: New York : Nova Science Publishers, [2023] | Series: Cardiology research and clinical developments | Includes bibliographical references and index. |
Identifiers: LCCN 2023043455 (print) | LCCN 2023043456 (ebook) | ISBN 9798891131750 (hardcover) | ISBN 9798891132504 (adobe pdf)
Subjects: LCSH: Pulmonary embolism. | Pulmonary embolism--Diagnosis. | Pulmonary embolism--Treatment. | Thromboembolism. | Thromboembolism--Diagnosis. | Thromboembolism--Treatment.
Classification: LCC RC776.P85 P826 2023 (print) | LCC RC776.P85 (ebook) | DDC 616.1/35--dc23/eng/20231026
LC record available at https://lccn.loc.gov/2023043455
LC ebook record available at https://lccn.loc.gov/2023043456

Published by Nova Science Publishers, Inc. † New York

Contents

Preface

Pulmonary embolism is one of the leading causes of cardiovascular mortality in the world and still one of the most underdiagnosed diagnosis in clinical practice. The serious acute and chronic consequences of pulmonary embolism and spending hours of clinical work in diagnosis and treatment of these patients give as a real view in to the pulmonary embolism burden. As clinicians we are facing everyday challenges in treatment of acute pulmonary embolism patients which are often very complex heterogeneous population. The improvements in diagnostic methods and revolution of anticoagulation therapy lead to decrease in-hospital mortality, especially in high risk patients. Despite these facts, the pulmonary embolism mortality remains still high. There are some incompletely answered question and grey zones in the pulmonary embolism treatment guidelines, that often make practical decisions difficult. Throughout our journey with many ongoing challenges we found ourselves longing for a reference book that will easily guide us thought the diagnosis and treatment of patients with acute pulmonary embolism. Treating these patients in intensive care unit inspired me to bring together great experts and enthusiasts in this field to create this book working together with the same goal. Exceptional support, inspiration and persistence of contributing authors, enable us to realize this project. We are extremely proud of the regional and European renowned pulmonary embolism and ultrasound experts we have been able to bring together, to cover everything from pathophysiology, risk stratification, treatment and prognosis in patients with deep vein thrombosis, acute pulmonary embolism as well as chronic thromboembolic pulmonary hypertension. This book also discusses the contemporary pulmonary embolism treatment approach in special patient population such as patients with cancer and pregnant women. The book is expected to help everyday clinical practice for physicians in the emergency departments, intensive care units and medical wards dealing with pulmonary embolism patients. We find it useful literature for diverse specialists included in the pulmonary embolism treatment (cardiologist, pulmologist, hematologist, intensive care physicians, interventional cardiologist and radiologists). We truly hope readers will find this book as educational and enjoyable to read as we have found inspiration in creating it.

Acknowledgments

We would like to thank our contributing authors for their hard work, enthusiasm and dedication for this book project, without whom this book would not have been possible. We would also like to thank to Dr. Tamara Kovacevic-Preradovic1, Dr. Aleksandar N. Neskovic2,3, Dr. Jelena M. Marinković4, Dr. Sandra M. Pekovic5, Dr Boris M. Dzudovic6,7, and Dr Jovan A. Matijasevic6,8 for their continued contribution in regional pulmonary embolism registry (REPER) and generously sharing their results, their dedication and mutual cooperation. Finally, we are truly grateful to our families, who have supported us unconditionally through the pathway of this project, their patience and understating. They have been our source of inspiration throughout our careers and supporters of our dreams.

1Clinic of Cardiology, Clinical Center Banja Luka, School of Medicine, University of Banja Luka, Republic of Srpska, Bosnia and Herzegovina, 2Department of Cardiology, Clinical Hospital Center Zemun, Serbia, 3School of Medicine Belgrade, University of Belgrade, Serbia, 4Institute for medical statistics School of Medicine, University of Belgrade, 5Institute for Pulmonary Diseases of Vojvodina, Serbia, 6School of Medicine, University of Defense, Belgrade, Serbia, 7Clinic of Emergency Internal Medicine, Military Medical Academy, Belgrade, Serbia, 8School of Medicine, University of Novi Sad, Serbia

Abbreviations

2D- two-dimensional echocardiography
3D – three-dimensional echocardiography
ABG - Arterial blood gas
AHF – acute heart failure
AP – supine
APL - antiphospholipid antibodies
APTT - Activated partial thrombin time
ART - assisted reproductive technology
BMI- body mass index
BNP - brain natriuretic peptic
BPA – balloon pulmonary angioplasty
CAT - carcinoma associated thromboembolism
CDT - catheter directed therapy
CHA2DS2-VASc - Chads vascular score
COMMAND VTE - JAPAN acute VTE registry
CP- cancer procoagulant factor
CrCl - creatinine clearance
CT- computer tomography
CTED - chronic thromboembolic pulmonary diseases
CTEPH - chronic thromboembolic pulmonary hypertension
cTn - cardiac troponin
CTPA - Computed Tomography Pulmonary Angiography
CURES - China pulmonary Thromboembolism Registry Study
CUS- Compression ultrasonography
DAPT - Dual antiplatelet therapy
DASH score - DASH Prediction Score for Recurrent venous thromboembolism
DECT - Dual energy CT
DM - diabetes mellitus
DOACS - direct oral anticoagulants

DSA - Digital subtraction angiography
DVT - deep vein thrombosis
ECG - Electrocardiography
ECMO - extracorporeal membrane oxygenation
EF - ejection fraction
FAC - functional area change
FH - family history
GFR - Glomerular filtration rate
HAS-BLED - HAS bleed score
HERDOO2 - clinical prediction rule for estimating the risk of recurrent venous thromboembolism
HIT - heparin induced thrombocytopenia
HR - heart rate
IBD - inflammatory bowel disease
ICOPER - International Cooperative Pulmonary Embolism Registry
IL-1 - interleukin-1
INR - international normalized ratio
IPAH – Idiopathic pulmonary arterial hypertension
IPER - Italian Pulmonary Embolism Registry
ISTH - International Society of Thrombosis and Hemostasis
ISTH - International Society of Thrombosis and Hemostasis
IVC - inferior vena cava
IVDU - intravenous drug user
IVF - in vitro fertilization
LMWH - low molecular heparin
LV - left ventricle
LVOT - left or right ventricular outflow tract
MP - microparticles
MRA - magnetic resonance angiography
MRI - magnetic resonance
MRPA - magnetic resonance pulmonary angiography
OHSS - ovarian hyper stimulation syndrome
PA - erect
PASP - pulmonary arterial systolic pressure
PEA – pulmonary enterectomy
PEBSI - Pulmonary Embolism Bleeding Score Index
PEITHO study - Pulmonary Embolism Thrombolysis trial
PERT - pulmonary embolism response team
PESI - Pulmonary embolism score index

PPH - primary postpartum hemorrhage
PVR - pulmonary vascular resistance
RA - right atrium
RAMs - risk-assessment models
RAP - right atrial pressure
REPER - Regional registry on pulmonary embolism
RHC – Right heart catheterization
RIETE - Computerized Registry of Patients with Venous Thromboembolism
RMPI – right myocardial performance index
RT- Randomized trial
RV - right ventricle
RVD - right ventricular dysfunction
RVSP - right ventricle systolic pressure
SBP - Systolic blood pressure
SLE - systemic lupus erythematosus
sPAP - systolic pulmonary artery pressure
SPECT - single photon computed tomography
STEMI - ST segment elevation myocardial infarction
TAPSE - tricuspid annular plane systolic excursion
TDI - Tissue Doppler Imaging
TEE - transesophageal echocardiography
99mTc MAA – Technetium 99m macro aggregated albumin
99mTc DTPA - Technetium 99m diethylenetriaminepentaacetic acid
TF- tissue factor
TNF- tumor necrosis factor
TNK - tenecteplase
tPA - tissue plasminogen activator
TR - tricuspid regurgitation
TTE - transthoracic echocardiography
UHF - unfractioned heparin
URL - upper confidence limit
V/Q scan - Ventilation perfusion scan
V-A ECMO - Venous-arterial extracorporeal membrane oxygenation
VEGF- vascular endothelial growth factor
VKA - Vitamin K antagonists
VTE - venous thromboembolism
VTI - velocity time integral
vTR - velocity of tricuspid regurgitation velocity
mGy – milli greys

vWF – factor von Wideband
VEGF - vascular endothelial growth factor

Chapter 1

Epidemiology, Pathophysiology, and Risk Factors for Pulmonary Embolism

Irena Mitevska*
University Cardiology Clinic, Clinical Center, Medical Faculty, Saints Cyril and Metodij University, Skopje, North Macedonia

Abstract

Pulmonary embolism (PE) is the third vascular cause of death and one of the most missed diagnoses in clinical practice. It is a potentially life-threatening condition that promotes a high level of clinical suspicion and often requires a fast diagnosis. PE and deep venous thrombosis (DVT) are part of the spectrum of venous thromboembolic disease (VTE). PE is associated with potential complications and high health-care costs, reduced quality of life, and increased patient disability. VTE is related to multiple acquired and inherited risk factors, advanced age, and in the last decades, carcinoma has surfaced as an important cause of PE (Howard et al., 2013). Contemporary knowledge about comorbidities and risk factors related to PE is mostly based on clinical studies and several large registries that closely reflect real-life PE patients. Clinical and hemodynamic repercussions of PE depend on the pulmonary embolism location, thrombus extension, degree of obstruction, previous cardiorespiratory disease, fast diagnosis, and proper patient treatment. Noninvasive evaluation of the right ventricular function and laboratory biomarkers are part of the patient's clinical assessment in the pathway of the pulmonary embolism trajectory. Understanding the pathophysiology of PE is very important for risk-stratifying patients and proper individual management. Pulmonary embolism is a global health care problem,

* Corresponding Author's Email: peovskai@yahoo.com.

In: Pulmonary Embolism
Editors: Irena Mitevska, Sonja Salinger, Marijan Bosevski et al.
ISBN: 979-8-89113-175-0

which requires continuous efforts to improve VTE awareness, fast diagnosis, effective implementation of acute phase treatment, and thromboprophylaxis measures.

Keywords: pulmonary embolism, epidemiology, pathophysiology

Introduction

Venous thromboembolism (VTE), is globally the third most frequent vascular cause of mortality, causing significant health burdens. Based on epidemiological studies, the annual incidence of PE rates ranges from 39 to 115 per 100,000 population, with frequency increasing in older individuals (Wendelboe et al., 2016). In the European Union, the incidence of PE is estimated to be around 350,000 individuals annually, or 15 to 60% per 1000 population per year (Wendelboe et al., 2016). Longitudinal studies have shown increasing annual PE incidence rates in recent decades, explained by patients aging, the high prevalence of chronic cardiovascular and respiratory diseases, autoimmune diseases, obesity, and carcinoma (John et al., 2015). Data from the World Health Organization (WHO) related to PE mortality in the 123 WHO member states report high PE death heterogeneity, with an age-standardized mortality of 0 to 24 deaths per 100,000 population annually, which indicates a significant underdiagnosis of PE (Barco et al., 2021). Current data indicates that up to 34% of PE patients die suddenly or within a few hours after the first symptoms, before the diagnosis is established and treatment is applied (Lehert et al., 2018, Barco et al., 2020). The projected PE case-fatality rate is approximately 6% after 30 days (Bach et al., 2016). The percentage of idiopathic VTE ranges from 25% to 40%. The long-term consequences of PE include the risk of recurrent episodes, and it is estimated that 20-25% of all patients have a recurrence within five years as well as the risk of chronic thromboembolic pulmonary hypertension (CTEPH). Scientific evidence has shown that intra-hospital and out of hospital early mortality is related to severity of PE and its hemodynamic repercussions, presence of right ventricular dysfunction (RVD), and subsequent hemodynamic compromise. Hemodynamically unstable patients are categorized as high-risk PE patients, based on the latest European Society of Cardiology (ESC) guidelines, with a mortality rate ranging from 35 to 58% in patients presenting with hypotension or shock (Konstantinides et al., 2020). Those patients represent 5% of all PE hospitalized patients. Approximately 40% of patients are categorized as intermediate risk patients based on early mortality risk stratification (Naess et al., 2007). An additional 55% of PE patients are assumed to be in the low-risk category, with a 30 day mortality risk less than 3% (Tapson et al., 2008).

Epidemiology of Venous Thromboembolism

Although PE is a major vascular cause of death with around ten million cases per year, PE-related intra-hospital death rates have decreased during the last decade, most probably indicating a greater prevalence of lower risk patients and improved PE management (Douglas et al., 2011). Between 5 and 10% of hospital deaths are a result of PE. Scientific data indicate particular PE vulnerability in obese patients, pregnant and postpartum women, and hospitalized patients with chronic cardiorespiratory disease and stroke for whom there are now scientific data and treatment guidelines. Cancer patients are at increased risk for PE, as well as chronic thromboembolic pulmonary hypertension (CTEPH). Improved VTE management with the use of direct oral anticoagulants (DOAC), invasive PE treatment with embolectomy, and thrombolytic catheters potentially reduce VTE mortality, long-term symptoms, and complications, which include post-thrombotic syndrome and chronic thromboembolic pulmonary hypertension (Sandblad et al., 2022). In the last three years, the COVID-19 pandemic significantly increased PE risk, especially among critically ill hospitalized patients (Kaiafa et al., 2022). The unique coagulopathy in COVID-19 patients is described as immune thrombosis with generalized endotheliopathy and *in situ* pulmonary vascular thrombosis with imbibition of inflammatory cells. The are many studies and several expert recommendations and guidance for treatment and thromboprophylaxis use in PE in patients with the COVID-19 infection in outpatient and hospital settings (Fauvel et al., 2020, Miró et al., 2021).

Age Distribution of Pulmonary Embolisms

Incidence rates of VTE in individuals over 70 years old are three times higher than those aged 45 to 69 years, which are three times higher compared to those aged 20 to 44 years (Cushman et al., 2007). The case fatality rate of a VTE event is 10% at 30 days, 15% within three months, and 20% by one year, but this also depends on patient risk and comorbidities (Heit et al., 2005).

Individuals over 80 years old have up to eight times higher incidence of PE, compared to younger patients.

Gender Differences in Pulmonary Embolism Prevalence and Mortality

There is evidence that younger women more frequently die of PE compared to younger male patients (Barrios et al., 2017). Those data point to the need for more intense prevention, diagnosis, and treatment of VTE during pregnancy and postpartum and analysis of factors predisposed to PE in younger women. The increasing prevalence of obesity and contraception use also increase PE risk in younger individuals of both genders who have higher mortality. In lower income countries, PE mortality is higher among older male individuals. Data report an overall 1.9-fold increase in PE risk in men compared with women without reproductive risk factors (Yoshikawa et al., 2019). Scientific data from several studies have found a higher PE-related mortality in women, possibly explained by higher rate of massive PEs in women. History of recent surgery, prolonged immobilization, and trauma have been significantly associated with the development of PE and are more prevalent in females compared to their male counterparts (38.4% women vs. 29.5% men; $p = 0.026$) (Pribish et al., 2020). Several trials have shown that women with acute PE are older by an average of 3.7 to 7 years and have higher brain natriuretic peptide (BNP) values compared to man with acute PE. Published studies have found higher and similar rates of malignancy in women compared to men (Kucher et al., 2003). The rate of VTE recurrences is similar for both genders, with similar cumulative three-year incidences of all-cause mortality.

Pathogenesis and Pathophysiology of Pulmonary Embolism

Pathogenesis

Most pulmonary emboli originate as thrombi in the deep veins of the lower extremities. The site of thrombosis is most often in the calf veins, femoropopliteal veins, and less frequently in the iliac veins. A smaller percentage of emboli arise from upper extremity veins and are typically associated with central venous catheters, intracardiac devices such as pacemakers and defibrillators, and malignancy or activity-related venous trauma. Pelvic vein DVTs can also cause pulmonary emboli, but they are generally associated with a predisposing factor such as pelvic infection, pelvic surgery, or pregnancy. Lower extremity central DVTs are most likely to embolize and cause PE (15–32% of the time), whereas upper extremity DVTs cause PE only 6% of the time (Turetz et al., 2018).

Pathophysiology

The most frequent pathophysiological mechanism of PE is detachment of emboli from their point of origin, usually in the lower extremity veins and they travel through the venous system, through the right sided chambers of the heart, and finally lodge in the pulmonary arterial system. The physiologic and clinical consequences of PE vary from asymptomatic to hemodynamic collapse and death. PE leads to gas exchange abnormalities and hypoxemia, but it is predominantly the hemodynamic consequences that are responsible for increased morbidity and mortality (Wood et al., 2002). An understanding of the pulmonary pathophysiology of PE is important in risk-stratifying patients and treatment choice with anticoagulation alone or the use of catheter-directed therapies (thrombolytics or mechanical thrombectomy), systemic thrombolytics, or surgical intervention (Laura et al., 2010).

Right ventricular (RV) failure due to acute pressure overload is considered the primary cause of death in severe PE. Pulmonary artery pressure (PAP) increases if >30-50% of the total cross-sectional area of the pulmonary arterial bed is occluded by a thrombus. PE-induced vasoconstriction, mediated by the release of thromboxane A2 and serotonin, contributes to the initial increase in pulmonary vascular resistance (PVR) after a PE event (Lyhne et al., 2020). The abrupt increase in PVR results in RV dilation, which alters the contractile properties of the RV myocardium via the Frank-Starling mechanism. The increase in RV pressure and volume leads to an increase in wall tension and myocyte stretch. Together with systemic vasoconstriction, these compensatory mechanisms increase PAP, improve flow through the obstructed pulmonary vascular bed, and thus temporarily stabilize systemic blood pressure (BP) (Greyson et al. 2000). However, the extent of immediate adaptation is limited, as a nonpreconditioned, thin-walled RV is unable to generate a mean PAP >40 mmHg. Prolongation of RV contraction time into early diastole in the left ventricle (LV) leads to leftward displacement of the interventricular septum (Ryan et al., 2015). As a result, LV filling is impeded in early diastole, and this may lead to a reduction in the cardiac output (CO) and contribute to systemic hypotension and hemodynamic instability (Lualdi et al., 1995). Excessive neurohumoral activation in PE can be the result of both abnormal RV wall tension and circulatory shock. The inflammatory response might explain the secondary hemodynamic destabilization that sometimes occurs 24-48 hours after acute PE, although early recurrence of PE may be an alternative explanation in some cases. Association between elevated circulating levels of biomarkers of myocardial injury and an adverse early outcome indicate that RV ischemia is of pathophysiological significance in the acute phase of PE (Janisset et al., 2022). RV infarction can further reduce contractile forces. Systemic hypotension is a critical element in this process, leading to impairment of the coronary driving pressure to the overloaded RV. The pathophysiologic consequences of acute PE are shown in Figure 1.

Acute RV failure is a critical determinant of clinical severity and outcome in acute PE. Clinical symptoms and signs of RV failure and hemodynamic instability indicate a high risk of early intra-hospital or 30-day mortality. The hemodynamic response to PE depends on the size of the embolus, location in the pulmonary circulation, coexistent cardiopulmonary disease, and neurohumoral effects (McIntyre et al., 1971). If obstruction is mild, peripheral vascular resistance (PVR) and pulmonary artery pressure remain normal by recruiting and distending pulmonary vessels.

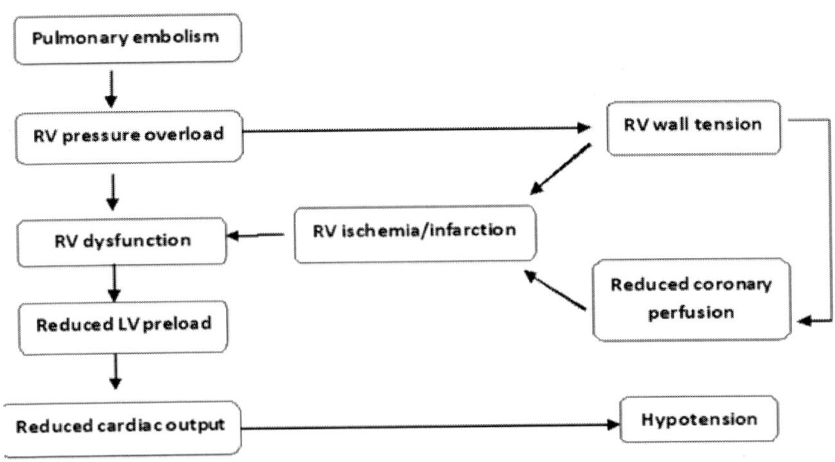

RV- right ventricle, LV – left ventricle

Figure 1. Pathophysiology of hemodynamic instability in acute pulmonary embolism.

At moderate levels of obstruction, pulmonary artery pressure and right atrial pressure increase. Initially, RV stroke volume and cardiac output are maintained by an increase in heart rate and contractility. In patients without prior chronic pulmonary disease, the maximal mean pulmonary artery pressure that can be generated even with >50% obstruction is ~ 40 mm Hg. An additional doubling of pulmonary artery pressure may occur in patients with prior pulmonary hypertension. Obstruction much beyond this will precipitate RV failure (Konstantinides et al., 2020). When the degree of obstruction exceeds 50 to 60%, the right heart dilates, RV wall tension increases, coronary perfusion pressure drops, RV ischemia and RV dysfunction develop, and cardiac output falls, leading to hypotension (Ventetuolo et al., 2014). While this pathological process evolves, most patients maintain a normal systemic arterial pressure for 12 to 48 hours and may give the impression of being hemodynamically stable. Then, often abruptly, pressor-resistant systemic arterial hypotension and cardiac arrest may ensue. With increased right ventricular wall stress, cardiac ischemia may develop, because increased right ventricular pressure compresses the right coronary artery, diminishes subendocardial perfusion, and limits myocardial oxygen supply. Elevations of troponin values are caused by right ventricular microinfarction, and right ventricular overload causes elevations of both pro-B-type natriuretic peptide and B-type natriuretic peptide (Lega et al., 2020).

Hypoxemia and Gas Exchange

Hypoxemia and an increase in the alveolar-arterial oxygen tension gradient are the most common gas exchange abnormalities in acute PE patients resulting in an increase in total dead space caused by obstruction of pulmonary artery by embolus. Ventilation perfusion mismatch follows, with redirection of the blood flow from obstructed pulmonary arteries to other gas exchange units, which can be potentiated by the presence of atelectasis (Overton et al., 1988). Arterial hypoxemia occurs when venous blood flows through lung gas exchange units, where the ratio of ventilation to capillary blood flow is low. In patients with acute PE, hypercapnia reflects massive embolism accompanied by marked increases in both anatomic and physiological dead space.

The following mechanisms are the major causes of hypoxemia in acute pulmonary embolism:

1. Ventilation perfusion mismatch. Overperfusion of non-embolized areas of the lung leads to insufficient ventilation and oxygenation of the extra blood flow.
2. Blood shunting occurs in collapsed and infarcted areas that are not ventilated but still obtain blood flow. In patients with a patent foramen ovale, increased right atrial pressure may open the foramen and cause right to left shunting at the atrial level, especially in cases with profound hypoxemia, which cannot be corrected by oxygen administration accompanied by hypercapnia.
3. Low mixed venous oxygen saturation that results from reduced cardiac output causes hypoxemia due to insufficient time for the severely desaturated blood to become fully saturated as it passes through the capillaries in the overperfused lung areas (Riedel et al., 2001).

Factors Related to Venous Thromboembolism

Three main factors influence the incidence of pulmonary embolism in the general population: (1) the prevalence of PE risk factors (2) the number and types of diagnostic methods, and (3) implementation of thromboprophylaxis recommendations and guidelines.

The etiology of PE has predominately focused on acquired and inherited causes of hypercoagulability; however; there are scientific data on associations between atherosclerosis and spontaneous intravascular venous thrombosis (Prandoni et al., 2003). Rudolph Virchow has identified the triad of risk factors that contribute to thrombosis, which include blood flow stasis, vascular damage, and hypercoagulability. All VTE risk factors affect these pathophysiologic processes. VTE is assumed to be a result of the interaction between patient-related risk factors and provoking most often temporary risk factors (Gjonbrataj et al., 2017). It is very important to categorize temporary and permanent risk factors for VTE for decision-making regarding the duration of anticoagulant therapy and assessment of the recurrence risk. The acquired VTE risk factors are categorized as strong (odds ratio >10), moderate (odds ratio 2–9), and weak (odds ratio <2). The incidence of unprovoked PE in adults is 25–40% (Heit et al., 2016).

Table 1. Acquired risk factors for pulmonary embolism

Acquired pulmonary embolism risk factors		
Weak (odds ratio M2)	**Medium (odds ratio 2-9)**	**Strong (odds ratio >10)**
Bed rest (>3 days)	Arthroscopic knee surgery	Fracture (hip or leg) Hip or knee replacement Major general surgery Major trauma
Extended immobility (air travel >8 hours) Increasing age (>40 years)	Central venous lines	Spinal cord injury
Laparoscopic surgery	Chemotherapy	Elevated level of factor VIII
Obesity	Congestive heart failure or respiratory failure, paralytic stroke, thrombophilia, hormone replacement therapy, or oral contraceptive therapy	
Pregnancy/antepartum	Malignancy	
Varicose veins	Pregnancy/postpartum; previous VTE	

Abbreviations: VTE- Venous thromboembolism

Acquired Risk Factors

Several prospective studies have reported an association between VTE and chronic peripheral arterial disease, hypertension, and dyslipidemia (Prandoni et al., 2007). This is explained by the fact that atherosclerosis is associated with higher platelet activation, blood coagulation, and increased fibrin turnover, which can all lead to thrombotic events. The list of acquired predisposing risk factors is shown in *Table 1*. The most common strong provoking risk factors for VTE are surgery, major trauma, spinal cord injury, lower-limb fractures, and joint replacements. Additionally, immobilization, bed rest over 72 hours, long air travel, cancer, oral contraceptives, pregnancy, smoking, postmenopausal hormone replacement therapy, obesity, and medical conditions, such as pneumonia, chronic respiratory disease, myocardial infarction, and congestive heart failure are factors that increase the risk for VTE (Mahmoodi et al., 2017). Several additional chronic medical conditions have been associated with increased PE risk, which include atherosclerosis, chronic kidney disease, nephrotic syndrome, polycythemia vera, paroxysmal nocturnal hemoglobinuria, Behcet's disease, rheumatoid arthritis, systemic lupus erythematosus, vasculitis, asthma, obstructive sleep apnea, polycystic ovary syndrome, and diabetes (Ageno et al., 2008). Infections including sepsis, tuberculosis, and more recently coronavirus disease are gaining importance. Respiratory infections and traumas explain higher prevalence of PE in the winter months. The risk of PE and obesity is correlated with the body mass index, which increases by 3.2-fold for those with a BMI ≥29 (61). Obesity is correlated with VTE, particularly in women (Hotoleanu et al., 2020). PE risks are also associated with flight duration. Scientific evidence has revealed a rate of 1.5 in one million individuals flying more than 5000 km and a rate of 4.8 in one million of those flying more than 10,000 km. Several conditions lead to hemoconcentration during air flight, such as dehydration, decreased oxygen pressure, and foot swelling, and these are assumed to induce venous stasis (Chandra et al., 2009).

Combined oral contraceptives (containing estrogen and progestogen) are associated with a two to sixfold increase in VTE risk in women (Grady et al., 1997). Inflammatory bowel disease, pneumonia, and urinary infections, as well as central venous lines, blood transfusions, and previous VTE are moderate risk factors. Older age, diabetes, and hypertension are among weaker PE predisposing factors (Ocak et al., 2013). Cancer is a well-established predisposing factor for VTE, which is gaining more importance with its increasing prevalence. The risk varies with different types of cancer, cancer activity, and the treatment used (Ay et al., 2010). The higher risk for VTE is related to pancreatic cancer, lung cancer, hematological malignancies, gastric cancer, and brain cancer (Khorana et al., 2008). Based on the RIETE Registry data, 45% of PE episodes have unknown risk, 23.4% are due to immobility, 22.5% of patients included had cancer, 10.7% had surgery, and 5.6% used hormone therapy (Tzoran et al., 2014).

Genetic Risk Factors

Thrombophilic disorders can be divided into loss-of-coagulation and gain-of-coagulation function disorders (Girolami et al., 2018). Loss-of-function disorders include deficiencies of the antithrombin, protein C, and protein S. They are less common than gain-of-function disorders, but may be more potent risk factors for thrombosis. Gain-of function disorders include factor V Leiden, the prothrombin 20210A variant, and elevation of procoagulant factors, such as factor VIII, von Willebrand factor, and factors V, VII, IX and XI. These disorders carry weaker risk for VTE (Girolam et al., 2018). Among the hereditary risk factors leading to a higher thrombotic risk, the strongest impact has an antithrombin deficiency, protein C and protein S deficiency, which represent only 15% of hereditary thrombophilia. Deficiencies in protein C, protein S, and antithrombin relatively increase the PE risk five to tenfold in affected individuals (Soare et al., 2008). Factor V Leiden is a more common mutation leading to hypercoagulability, and it is associated with a fivefold increased risk of VTE with heterozygotes and a tenfold risk with homozygotes. Finally, the prothrombin gene mutation can be detected in 7% of patients with VTE and increases the risk of thrombosis threefold (Rosendaal et al., 1995).

Homozygote mutation for factor V Leiden is the most frequent hereditary thrombophilia, causing the etiology in 20% of patients with thrombosis. Similarly, hyperhomocysteinemia and a mutation in the prothrombin gene were shown to cause hereditary thrombophilia. The individuals with heterozygous factor Leiden mutation have a three to sixfold increased VTE risk (den Heijer et al., 2005). Factor V Leiden is present in 10-50% of the cases with VTE. Factor II G20210A mutation increases the plasma prothrombin level, which results in a predisposition to thrombosis. This mutation was detected in 1-3% of the general population and 6-18% of patients with VTE. A high FVIII level was reported to increase the VTE risk approximately fivefold compared to individuals with a normal level (Vince et al., 2012). Venous thrombosis often occurs when multiple risk factors, including genetic and environmental, are present at the same time. It is estimated that women heterozygous for factor V Leiden using oral contraceptives have a 34-fold increased relative risk for PE (Spannagl et al., 2000). Antiphospholipid syndrome is characterized by recurrent venous or arterial thrombosis with VTE occurring in one-third of patients (Shi et al., 2022). The risk of VTE is 5 to 8% higher in patients who carry lupus anticoagulant or anti-β_2-glycoprotein I antibodies. The most common inherited risk factors for PE are described in Tablc 2.

Hyperhomocysteinemia

Hyperhomocysteinemia is the only hereditary cause of thrombophilia that has been proven to lead to arterial and venous thrombosis. It is believed to trigger the development of thrombosis by affecting the endothelial cells and causing the formation of reactive oxygen forms, smooth muscle cells proliferation, increasing collagen production, and tissue factor production in the monocytes, as well as increasing the synthesis of thromboxane in the platelet.

Hyperhomocysteinemia is associated with a two to fourfold increased thrombotic risk. Plasma homocysteine concentration is affected by genetic and acquired factors and thus known as the mixed risk factor (Tsai et al., 2003). Vitamin B12, vitamin B6 and folate deficiency, advanced age, chronic renal failure, and malnutrition involving anti-folic drug use represent acquired factors in hyperhomocysteinemia. Gene defects in two enzymes involved in the intracellular metabolism, methyl tetrahydrofolate reductase (MTHFR) and cystathionine B-synthase (CBS) result in hyperhomocysteinemia and enzyme deficiency. Hyperhomocysteinemia is not defined as a genetic abnormality for VTE but as an independent risk factor (Phillips et al., 1997). Additional inherited thrombophilia risk factors are dysfibrinogenemia, Factor XII deficiency, and non-O blood group.

Iatrogenic Causes of Pulmonary Embolism

Several drugs have been associated with increased risk of VTE, which include contraceptive medications as the most important, especially in young women, and hormone replacement therapy in postmenopausal women. Other drugs reported as a risk factor for VTE include systemic glucocorticoids, tamoxifen, testosterone, heparin-induced thrombocytopenia, and antidepressants. Intravenous drug use has been associated with deep vein thrombosis due to local trauma and irritation of femoral veins in the lower extremities through injections by drug abusers (Shannon et al., 2017).

Table 2. Inherited risk factors for pulmonary embolism

Inherited pulmonary embolism risk factors		
Weak	**Medium**	**Strong**
Hyperhomocystinemia	Mutation of factor V Leiden	Deficit of AT III, protein C, protein S
	Mutation of prothrombin (factor II) gene (prothrombin 202110A); Deficiency of factors VII, XII, IX	Insufficient anticoagulant pathways, such as tissue factor pathway inhibitors, thrombomodulin. and endothelial protein C receptor
	Blood group (non-O)	Elevated level of factor VIII
	C to T variation at position of 10034 in the fibrinogen gamma chain	

Venous Thromboembolism Recurrence Risk

Patients with VTE have frequent recurrence episodes. Approximately 30% of patients with VTE experience recurrence within ten years (Christiansen et al., 2010). The risk of a first VTE recurrence varies according to the time from the first event, and is highest in the first 6 to 12 months. Scientific data has found a significant correlation between the type of initial and recurrent events. The most frequently recurring episodes after the initial PE are repetitive PE, and this similarly occurs after the first proximal DVT. Based on a study of inhabitants of Olmsted County, Minnesota, the cumulative incidence of the first VTE recurrence was estimated at 5.2% at 30 days, 8.3% at 90 days, 12.9% at one year, 16.6% at two years, 22.8% at five years (Heit et al., 2000). Secondary prophylaxis is very effective in preventing VTE recurrence; however, duration and type of acute treatment does not affect the recurrence rate after the initial three months of prophylactic anticoagulation therapy. Independent predictors of recurrent VTE episodes include male sex, increasing patient age, previous stroke, obesity, active cancer, idiopatic VTE with persistent elevation of D-dimers after anticoagulation therapy, residual vein thrombosis, and thrombophilias (deficiency of antithrombin III, protein C, or protein S, hyperhomocysteinemia, homozygous factor V Leiden mutations) (Heit et al., 2020). Factors associated with increased risk of VTE recurrence in patients with active cancer are cancer site (pancreatic, ovarian cancer, brain, lung, myeloproliferative, or myelodysplastic disorders), advanced cancer stage, cancer stage progression, and immobility (Louzada ML et al., 2011). From other sites, provoked risk factors for PE are associated with reduced risk of recurrence.

In women, pregnancy or puerperium, oral contraception, hormone therapy, and gynecological surgery at the VTE are associated with reduced risk of recurrence (Goldhaber at al., 1997, Heit et al., 2005). Patients with sub-segmental and more proximal PE have a similar three-month recurrence risk (Albertsen et al., 2018). There are several VTE recurrence prediction algorithms in patients with idiopathic non-provoked or cancer-associated VTE. In the HERDOO2 risk model, no predictors of a reduced risk of recurrent thrombotic events were found in men with idiopathic VTE. To the contrary, women with incident VTE who had a score of ≤1 had a significantly lower risk of recurrence VTE episodes than those with >1 (Rodger et al., 2017). The risk factors include older age (≥65 years), obesity, increased D-dimer values prior to stopping warfarin therapy, and presence of post-thrombotic syndrome. The Vienna prediction model includes male sex, incident VTE type (PE and/or proximal DVT versus isolated calf DVT), and increased D-dimer levels as predictors of recurrence after idiopathic VTE. In the DASH prediction model, persistently increased D-dimer level after termination of anticoagulation therapy, age <50 years, male sex, and VTE unrelated to hormonal therapy in women predicted an increased risk of recurrence after an idiopathic incident VTE (Tosetto et al., 2017). Older age is associated with a higher recurrence risk among women in the HERDOO2 model; younger age is associated with a higher risk in men and women in the DASH model; and age is not a predictor of recurrence in the Vienna model (Eichinger et al., 2010). Based on these scores, approximately 50% of patients with idiopathic VTE and a low prediction score could avoid secondary prophylaxis. Among patients with active cancer and VTE, female sex, cancer site (lung) and previous VTE are high-risk predictors of VTE recurrence, and cancer site (breast) and stage I are low-risk predictors in patients receiving anticoagulation therapy (Cheng et al., 2014).

Conclusion

Pulmonary embolism (PE) remains an important cause of cardiovascular burden, although the mortality rate is decreasing. Several inherited and acquired or provoked factors are involved in the etiology of PE, which are important to determine, since they are related to the risk of PE recurrence. PE severity determines pathophysiological and hemodynamic consequences. Clinical outcomes are closely related to the severity of pulmonary artery obstruction, increased pulmonary vascular resistance, right ventricle pressure load, and right ventricular dysfunction. Knowledge of etiology and pathophysiological consequences of PE are important for acute and long-term patient management.

References

Ageno, W., Becattini, C., Brighton, T., Selby, R., and Kamphuisen, P. W. (2008). Cardiovascular risk factors and venous thromboembolism: a meta-analysis. *Circ.*, 117, 93–102.

Albertsen, I. E., Nielsen, P. B., Søgaard, M., Goldhaber S. Z., Overvad. T. F., Rasmussen, L. H., and Larsen, T. B. (2018). Risk of recurrent venous thromboembolism: a Danish nationwide cohort study. *Am J Med.*, 131(9), 1067-1074.

Ay, C., Dunkler, D., Marosi, C., Chiriac, A. L., Vormittag, R., Simanek, R., Quehenberger, P., Zielinski, C., and Pabinger, I. (2010). Prediction of venous thromboembolism in cancer patients. *Blood.*, 116, 5377–5382.

Bach, A. G., Taute, B. M., Baasai, N., Wienke, A., Meyer, H. J., Schramm, D., and Surov, A. (2016). 30-day mortality in acute pulmonary embolism: prognostic value of clinical scores and anamnestic features. *PLoS One.*, 11(2), e0148728.

Barco, S., Mahmoudpour, S. H., Valerio, L., Klok, F. A., Münzel, T., Middeldorp, S., Ageno, W., Cohen, A. T., Hunt B. J., and Konstantinides, S. V. (2020). Trends in mortality related to pulmonary embolism in the European Region, 2000–15: analysis of vital registration data from the WHO Mortality Database. *Lancet Respir Med.*, 8, 277-287.

Barco, S., Valerio, L., Gallo, A., Turatti, G., Mahmoudpour. S. H., Ageno, W., Castellucci, L. A., Maus, G. C., Ddungu, H., De Paula, E. V., Dumantepe, M., Goldhaber, S. Z., Klok, F. A., Kucher, N., McLintock, C., Áinle F., Simioni, P., Spirk, D., Spyropoulos, A. C., Urano, T., Zhai, Z. G., Hunt, B. J., and Konstantinides, S. V. (2021 July). Global reporting of pulmonary embolism–related deaths in the World Health Organization mortality database: vital registration data from 123 countries. *Res Pract Thromb Haemost.*, 5(5), e12520.

Chandra, D., Parisini, E., and Mozaffarian, D. (2009). Meta-analysis: travel and risk for venous thromboembolism. *Ann. Intern. Med.*, 151, 180–190.

Chee, C. E., Ashrani, A. A., Marks, R. S., Petterson, T. M., Bailey, K. R., Melton, L. J., and Heit, J. A. (2014). Predictors of venous thromboembolism recurrence and bleeding among active cancer patients: a population-based cohort study. *Blood.*, June 19, 123(25), 3972–3978.

Christiansen, S. C., Lijfering, W. M., Helmerhorst, F. M., Rosendaal, F. R., and Cannegieter, S. C. (2010). Sex difference in risk of recurrent venous thrombosis and the risk profile for a second event. *J Thromb Haemost*, 8, 2159–68.

Cushman, M. (2007 Apr). Epidemiology and Risk Factors for Venous Thrombosis. *Semin Hematol.*, 44(2), 62–69.

Barrios, D., Morillo, R., Guerassimov, I., Barbero, E., Morreale, H. E., Cohen, A. T., Becattini, C., Tapson, V., Yusen, R., and Jimenez, D. (2017). Sex differences in the characteristics and short-term prognosis of patients presenting with acute symptomatic pulmonary embolism. *PLoS One*, 12, e 0187648.

Den Heijer, M., Lewington, S., and Clarke, R. (2005). Homocysteine, MTHFR and risk of venous thrombosis: a meta-analysis of published epidemiological studies. *J Thromb Haemost.*, 3, 292–299.

Dentali, F., Ageno, W., Pomero, F., Fenoglio, L., Squizzato, A., and Bonzini, M. (2016). Time trends and case fatality rate of in-hospital treated pulmonary embolism during 11 years of observation in Northwestern Italy. *Thromb Haemost.*, 115, 399-405.

Douketis, J. D., Foster, G. A., Crowther, M. A., Prins, M. H., and Ginsberg, J. S. (2000). Clinical risk factors and timing of recurrent venous thromboembolism during the initial 3 months of anticoagulant therapy. *Arch Intern Med.*, 160, 3431–3436.

Eichinger, S., Heinze, G., Jandeck, L. M., and Kyrle, P. A. (2010). Risk assessment of recurrence in patients with unprovoked deep vein thrombosis or pulmonary embolism: the Vienna prediction model. *Circ.*, 121, 1630–1636.

Fauvel, C., Weizman, O., Trimaille, A., Mika, D., Pommier, T., and Pace, N. (2020 Jul 1). Pulmonary embolism in COVID-19 patients: a French multicentre cohort study. *Eur Heart J.*, 41(32), 3058-3068.

Girolam, A., Cosi, E., Ferrari, S., Lombardi, A., and Fabris, F. (2018 May). Thrombotic and hemorrhagic conditions due to a gain of function of coagulation proteins: a special type of clotting disorders. *Clin Appl Thromb Hemost.*, 24(4), 560-565.

Gjonbrataj, E., Kim, J. N., Gjonbrataj, J., Jung, H. I., Kim, H. J., and Won, I. C. (2017 Jan). Risk factors associated with provoked pulmonary embolism. *Korean J Intern Med.*, 32(1), 95–101.

GliseSandblad, K., Rosengren, A., Sörbo, J., Jern, S., and Hansson, P. O. (2022 May). Pulmonary embolism and deep vein thrombosis-comorbidities and temporary provoking factors in a register-based study of 1.48 million people. *Res Pract Thromb Haemost.*, 6(4), e12714.

Goldhaber, S. Z., Grodstein, F., Stampfer, M. J., Manson, J. E., Colditz, G. A., Speizer, F. E., Willett, W. C., and Hennekens, C. H. (1997). A prospective study of risk factors for pulmonary embolism in women. *JAMA.*, 277, 642-645.

Grady, D., Hulley, S. B., and Furberg, C. (1997). Venous thromboembolic events associated with hormone replacement therapy. *JAMA.*, 278, 477.

Greyson, C., Xu, Y., Lu, L., and Schwartz, G. G. (2000). Right ventricular pressure and dilation during pressure overload determine dysfunction after pressure overload. *Am J Physiol Heart Circ Physiol*, 278, H1414–20.

Heit, J. A., Kobbervig, C. E., James, A. H., Petterson, T. M, Bailey, K. R., and Melton, L. J. (2005). Trends in the incidence of venous thromboembolism during pregnancy or postpartum: a 30-year population-based study. *Ann Intern Med.*, 143(10), 697–706.

Heit, J. A., Spencer, F. A., and White, R. H. (2016). The epidemiology of venous thromboembolism. *J Thromb Thrombolysis.*, 41, 3–14.

Heit, J. A., Mohr, D. N., Silverstein, M. D., Petterson, T. M., O'Fallon, W. M., and Melton, L. J. (2000). Predictors of recurrence after deep vein thrombosis and pulmonary embolism: a population-based cohort study. *Arch Intern Med.*, 160, 761–768.

Heit, J. A. (2015 Aug). Epidemiology of venous thromboembolism. *Nat Rev Cardiol.*, 12(8), 464–474.

Heit, J. A. (2005). Venous thromboembolism: disease burden, outcomes and risk factors. *J Thromb Haemost.*, 3, 1611–1617.

Hotoleanu, C. (2020 Apr). Association between obesity and venous thromboembolism. *Med Pharm Rep.*, 93(2), 162–168.

Howard, L. S., and Hughes, R. J. (2013). NICE guideline: Management of venous thromboembolic diseases and role of thrombophilia testing. *Thorax.*, 68, 391–393.

Janisset, L., Castan, M., Poenou, G., Lachand, R., Mismetti, P., Viallon. T., and Bertoletti, L. (2022 Apr). Cardiac biomarkers in patients with acute -pulmonary embolism. *Medicina (Kaunas).*, 58(4), 541.

Kaiafa, G., Savopoulos, C., Karlafti, E., Pantazi, K., Paramythiotis, D., Thomaidou, E., Daios, S., Ztriva, E., Michalis Gionis, Fyntanidou, V., Argiriadou H., and Didangelos, T. (2022 Oct). Coagulation profile of COVID-19 patients. *Life (Basel).*, 20, 12(10), 1658.

Khorana, A. A., Kuderer, N. M., Culakova, E., Lyman, G. H., and Francis, C. W. (2008). Development and validation of a predictive model for chemotherapy-associated thrombosis. *Blood.*, 111, 4902–4907.

Konstantinides, S. V., Meyer, G., Becattini, C., Bueno, H., Geersing, G. J., Harjola, V. P., Huisman, M. V., Humbert, M., Jennings, C. S., Jiménez, D., Kucher, N., Lang, I. M., Lankeit, M., Lorusso, R., Mazzolai, L., Meneveau, N., Áinle, F. N., Prandoni, P., Pruszczyk, P., Righini, M., Torbicki, A., Belle, E. V., and Zamorano, J. L. (2020 Jan 21). ESC Scientific Document Group. ESC Guidelines for the diagnosis and management of acute pulmonary embolism developed in collaboration with the European Respiratory Society (ERS). *Eur Heart J.*, 41(4), 543-603.

Kopcke, D., Harryman, O., Benbow, E. W., Hay, C., and Chalmers, N. (2011 Aug). Mortality from pulmonary embolism is decreasing in hospital patients. *J R Soc Med.*, 104(8), 327–331.

Kucher, N., Printzen, G., and Goldhaber, S. Z. (2003 May 27). Prognostic role of brain natriuretic peptide in acute pulmonary embolism. *Circ*, 107(20), 2545-7.

Lega, J. C., Lacasse, Y., Lakhal, L., and Provencher, S. (2009). Natriuretic peptides and troponins in pulmonary embolism: a meta-analysis. *Thorax*, 64, 869–875.

Lehnert, P., Lange, T., Møller, C. H., Olsen, P. S., and Carlsen, J. (2018). Acute pulmonary embolism in a national Danish cohort: increasing incidence and decreasing mortality. *Thromb Haemost.*, 118(3), 539-546.

Louzada, M. L., Majeed, H., Dao, V., and Wells, P. S. (2011). Risk of recurrent venous thromboembolism according to malignancy characteristics in patients with cancer-associated thrombosis: a systematic review of observational and intervention studies. *Blood Coagul Fibrinolysis.*, 22, 86–91.

Lualdi, J. C., and Goldhaber, S. Z. (1995). Right ventricular dysfunction after acute pulmonary embolism: pathophysiologic factors, detection, and therapeutic implications. *Am Heart J.*, 130(06), 1276–1282.

Lyhne, M. D., Kline, J. A., Nielsen-Kudsk, J. E., and Andersen, A. (2020 Jan-Mar). Pulmonary vasodilation in acute pulmonary embolism – a systematic review. *Pulm Circ.*, 10(1), 2045894019899775.

Mahmoodi, B. K., Cushman, M., Næss, I. A., Allison, M. A., Bos, W. J., Brækkan, S. K., Cannegieter, S. C. Gansevoort, R. T., Gona, P. N., Hammerstrøm. J., Hansen, J. B., Heckbert, S., Holst, A. G., Lakoski, S. G., Lutsey P. L., Manson, J. E., Martin, L. W., Matsushita, K., Meijer, K., Overvad, K., Prescott, E., Puurunen, M., Rossouw, J. E., Sang, Y., Severinsen, M. T., Berg, J. T., Folsom, A. R., and Zakai, N. A. (2017 Jan 3). Association of traditional cardiovascular risk factors with venous thromboembolism: an individual participant data meta-analysis of prospective studies. *Circ.*, 135(1), 7–16.

McIntyre, K. M., and Sasahara, A. A. (1971 Sept). The hemodynamic response to pulmonary embolism in patients without prior cardiopulmonary disease. *Am J Cardiol.*, 28(3), 288-94.

Miró, O., Jiménez, S., Mebazaa, A., Freund, Y., Burillo-Putze, G., and Martín, A. (2021). Pulmonary embolism in patients with COVID-19: incidence, risk factors, clinical characteristics, and outcome. *Eur Heart J.*, 42, 3127–3142.

Naess, I. A., Christiansen, S. C., Romundstad, P., Cannegieter, S. C., Rosendaal, F. R., and Hammerstrøm, J. (2007). Incidence and mortality of venous thrombosis: a population-based study. *J Thromb Haemost.*, 5(04), 692–699.

Ocak, G., Vossen, C. Y., Verduijn, M., Dekker, F. W., Rosendaal, F. R., Cannegieter, S. C., and Lijfering, W. M. (2013 Jan). Risk of venous thrombosis in patients with major illnesses: results from the MEGA study. *J Thromb Haemost.*, 11(1), 116-23.

Overton, D. T., and Bocka, J. J. (1988). The alveolar-arterial oxygen gradient in patients with documented pulmonary embolism. *Arch Intern Med.*, 148(07), 1617–1619.

Phillips, M. D. (1997). Interrelated risk factors for venous thromboembolism. *Circ.*, 95, 1749–1751.

Prandoni, P. (2007). Venous thromboembolism and atherosclerosis: is there a link? *J Thromb Haemost.*, 5(Suppl 1), 270–5.

Pribish, A., Beyer, S., Krawisz, A., Weinberg, I., Carroll, B. J., and Secemsky, E. A. (2020). Sex differences in presentation, management, and outcomes among patients hospitalized with acute pulmonary embolism. *Vasc Med*, 25, 541-48.

Price, L. C., Wort S. J., Finney, S. J., Marino P. S., and Brett S. J. (2010). Pulmonary vascular and right ventricular dysfunction in adult critical care: current and emerging options for management: a systematic literature review. *Crit Care.*, 14(5), R169.

Riedel, M. (2001). Acute pulmonary embolism 1: pathophysiology, clinical presentation, and diagnosis. *Heart*, 85, 229–240.

Rodger, M. A., Le Gal, G, Anderson D. R., Schmid J., Pernod G., Kahn S. R., Righini, M., Mismetti P., Kearon C., Meyer G., Elias A., Ramsay T., Ortel T. L., Menno V., Huisman, M. V., and Kovacs, M. J. (2017). REVERSE II study investigators. Validating the HERDOO2 rule to guide treatment duration for women with unprovoked venous thrombosis: multinational prospective cohort management study. *BMJ.*, 356, j1065.

Rosendaal, F. R., Koster, T., Vandenbroucke, J. P., and Reitsma, P. H. (1995). High risk of thrombosis in patients homozygous for factor V Leiden (activated protein C resistance). *Blood.*, 85, 1504–8.

Ryan, J. J., Huston, J., Kutty, S., Hatton, N. D., Bowman, L., Tian, L., Herr, J. E., Johri, A. M., and Archer, S. L. (2015 Apr). Right ventricular adaptation and failure in pulmonary arterial hypertension. *Can J Cardiol.*, 31(4), 391–406.

Shannon, M., Fernando, P. M., Pena, M., and Pena E. (2017). Iatrogenic pulmonary air embolism. *CMAJ*, August 21, 189 (33), E1069.

Shi, M., Gao, W., Jin, W., Zhu, J., Liu, Y., Wang, T., and Li, C. (2022). Antiphospholipid syndrome-related pulmonary embolism: clinical characteristics and early recognition. *Front Cardiovasc Med.*, 9, 872523.

Soare, A. M. (2018 May). Deficiencies of proteins C, S and antithrombin and activated protein C resistance–their involvement in the occurrence of arterial thromboses. *Clin Appl Thromb Hemost.*, 24(4), 560–565.

Spannagl, M., Heinemann, L. A., and Schramm, W. (2000 June). Are factor V Leiden carriers who use oral contraceptives at extreme risk for venous thromboembolism? *Eur J Contracept Reprod Health Care.*, 5(2), 105-12.

Stevens, S. M., Woller, S. C., Kreuziger, L. B., Bounameaux, H., Doerschug, K., Geersing, G. J., Huisman, M. V., Kearon, C., King, S. C., Knighton, A. J., Lake, E., Murin, S.,

Vintch. J. R. E., Wells, P. S., and Moores, L. K. (2021 Dec). Antithrombotic therapy for VTE disease: second update of the CHEST guideline and expert panel report. *Chest*, 160(6), e545-e608.

Tapson, V. F. (2008). Acute pulmonary embolism. *N Engl J Med.*, 358(10), 1037–1052.

Tosetto, A., Testa, S., Martinelli, I., Poli, D., Cosmi, B., Lodigiani, C., Ageno, W., De Stefano, V., Falanga, A., Nichele, I., Paoletti, O., Bucciarelli, P., Antonucci, E., Legnani, C., Banfi, E., Dentli, F., Bartolomeni F., Barcella, L., and Palareti, G. (2017 Oct). External validation of the DASH prediction rule: a retrospective cohort study. *J Thromb Haemost*, 15 (10), 1963-1970.

Tsai, A. W., Cushman, M., Tsai, M. Y., Heckbert, S. R., Rosamond, W. D., Aleksic, N., Yanez, N. D., Psaty, B. M., and Folsom, A. R. (2003). Serum homocysteine, thermolabile variant of methylene tetrahydrofolate reductase (MTHFR), and venous thromboembolism: longitudinal investigation of thromboembolism etiology (LITE) *Am J Hematol.*, 72, 192.

Turetz, M., Sideris, A. T., Friedman, O. A., Triphathi, N., and Horowitz, J. M. (2018 June). Pulmonary embolism epidemiology, pathophysiology, and natural history of pulmonary embolism. *Semin Intervent Radiol.*, 35(2), 92–98.

Tzoran, I., Brenner, B., Papadakis, M., Di Micco, P., and Monreal, M. (2014 Oct). VTE Registry: What can be learned from RIETE? *Rambam Maimonides Med J.*, 5(4), e003.

Ventetuolo, C. E., and Klinger, J. R. (2014 June). Management of acute right ventricular failure in the intensive care unit. *Ann Am Thorac Soc.*, 11(5), 811–822.

Vince, P., Jenkins, P. V., Rawley, O., Owen, P., and Donnell, J. S. (2012 June). Elevated factor VIII levels and risk of venous thrombosis. *B J Haem.*, 157(6).

Wendelboe, A. M., and Raskob, G. E. (2016). Global burden of thrombosis: epidemiologic aspects. *Circ Res.*, 118, 13401347.

Wood, K. E. (2002). Major pulmonary embolism: review of a pathophysiologic approach to the golden hour of hemodynamically significant pulmonary embolism. *Chest.*, 121(03), 877–905.

Yoshikawa, Y., Yamashita, Y., Morimoto, T., Amano, H., Takase, T., Hiramori, S., Kim, K., Maki, O., Akao, M,, Kobayashi, Y., Toyofuku, M., Izumi, T., Tada, T., Chen, P. M., Murata, K., Tsuyuki, Y., Saga, S., Sasa, T., Sakamoto, J., Kinoshita, K., Togi, K., Mabuchi, H., Takabayashi, K., Shiomi, H., Kato, T., Makiyama, T., Ono, K., and Kimura, T. (2019). COMMAND VTE Registry investigators. Sex differences in clinical characteristics and outcomes of patients with venous thromboembolism – from the COMMAND VTE Registry. *Circ J*, 83, 1581–89.

Chapter 2

The Diagnosis of Acute Pulmonary Embolism: The Integration of Clinical Scores, Biomarkers and Imaging Modalities

Irena Mitevska, PhD
University Cardiology Clinic, Clinical Center, Medical Faculty, Saints Cyril and Metodij University, Skopje, North Macedonia

Abstract

Pulmonary embolism (PE), one of the major causes of vascular mortality, necessitates prompt diagnosis and risk stratification in order to use proper management and reduce patient mortality. High clinical suspicion and the use of clinical probability based on several well-established scores (Wells and Geneva scores) are important in not overlooking PE diagnoses. The latest clinical guidelines include simple management algorithms and decision pathways. Clinical scores, biomarkers, and imaging modalities lead to improved diagnostic accuracy, standardized risk stratification, and individualized patient approaches. These diagnostic algorithms are based on the evaluation of pretest probability, laboratory biomarkers, D-dimer measurement, and imaging modalities that include echocardiography and computed tomography pulmonary angiography. All algorithms and scores allow for a safe and cost-effective approach to establishing proper diagnoses in the majority of patients with suspected PE. This chapter not only summarizes the clinical signs and symptoms of PE, PE probability scores, the diagnostic approach, and risk stratification, but also points to the diagnostic challenges of PE. The clinical importance of subsegmental PE is also addressed in this chapter. Differential diagnoses of PE and other acute emergency diseases is an important part of the clinical reasoning when

In: Pulmonary Embolism
Editors: Irena Mitevska, Sonja Salinger, Marijan Bosevski et al.
ISBN: 979-8-89113-175-0

evaluating patients with suspected PE. The priority goal of fast diagnosis is underlined along with all steps to obtain proper decisions while using an individualized approach.

Keywords: diagnosis, pulmonary embolism, imaging, biomarkers

Introduction

Acute PE is one of the most overlooked, underdiagnosed and potentially fatal emergency clinical conditions. Pulmonary embolism has a wide clinical presentation, from asymptomatic subsegment PE to life-threatening massive PE causing obstructive shock (Righini et al., 2017). The mechanism of pulmonary embolism (PE) is the occlusion of pulmonary artery branches caused by thrombi that typically originate in the large veins of the legs or pelvis. Initial clinical assessments, which includes hemodynamic stability, PESI scores, right ventricular function and high-sensitive Troponin I are essential for patient risk profile gradation, treatment, and prognosis (Konstantinides et al., 2018). Early hospital discharge with anti-coagulation treatment may be considered in patients with low risk PE. Computed tomographic pulmonary angiography (CTPA) is the most common imaging method that enables us to confirm the diagnosis of acute PE, but it also identifies right ventricular dysfunction or additional causes of patient instability. V/Q scintigraphy should be considered for patients with contraindications to iodinated contrast and normal chest radiographs, especially in younger women. Compression ultrasonography of the lower extremities, should be considered for patients suspected of acute PE with signs of lower extremity deep venous thrombosis or for patients with negative CTPA or V/Q scan with discordant clinical probability (Burns et al., 2012). Echocardiography is a basic method for assessment of hemodynamic repercussion of PE, RV function, and pulmonary hypertension, as well as assessment of the left ventricular function and potential complications (Dabbouseh et al., 2019). Biomarkers are part of the clinical assessment that modify patient risk. Incorporation of the full spectrum of the relevant clinical data, PE probability scores, biomarkers, and imaging data enables a fast diagnosis and proper management decisions that might modify a patient's prognosis.

Clinical Symptoms

Acute PE is characterized by clinical signs and symptoms that are nonspecific, and this is the cause of frequently missed diagnoses of pulmonary embolisms. Symptoms and signs vary according to the thrombus location, size, and extent, the degree of humoral response, and the cardiopulmonary reserve of the patient. These established facts imply high PE suspicion incorporating all clinical, ECG, imaging and biomarker data (Pollack et al., 2011). Some of the most frequent symptoms in suspected PE patients are dyspnea, syncope, chest pain, hemoptysis, palpitations, and shortness of breath. PE should be considered in patients with onset of significant, unexplained tachycardia and dyspnea, often with altered mental status, especially in elderly patients (Miniati et al., 1999). An important form of clinical presentation is hemodynamic instability, which indicates central and extensive PE with reduced right ventricular (RV) function and severely compromised hemodynamic reserve. Syncope is associated with a higher prevalence of hemodynamic instability and RV dysfunction (Barco et al., 2018).

Based on the results of several studies, acute PE may be frequently found in patients presenting with syncope even in the presence of alternative disease options. In some patients, PE may be asymptomatic or discovered incidentally during diagnostic workup for another disease. This occurs most frequently in patients with subsegmenal PE and small peripheral PE. Dyspnea may be acute and severe in central PE. In patients with established cardiorespiratory disease including heart failure, worsening dyspnea may be the only symptom indicative of PE. Chest pain is usually caused by pleural irritation due to more distal emboli associated with pulmonary infarction. In central and more severe PE, chest pain may have anginal characteristics, most possibly reflecting RV ischemia, which requires a different diagnosis from an acute coronary syndrome or aortic dissection. In addition to clinical symptoms, information of the predisposing factors for VTE and comorbidities is important in assessing the PE clinical probability, which increases with the number of predisposing risk factors. However, it is important to note that in approximately 40% of patients with PE, there are no predisposing factors that can be identified (Rodríguez-Núñez et al., 2020). Gas analyses often show hypoxemia and hypocapnia, with a normal alveolararterial oxygen gradient. Chest X-rays are frequently abnormal, and the findings are usually nonspecific in PE; however, these may be useful for excluding other causes of dyspnea or chest pain.

PE should be considered in the differential diagnosis of patients suspected of having the following conditions:

- Acute chest pain (acute coronary syndrome and aortic dissection)
- Heart failure
- Chronic respiratory failure (emphysema)
- Chronic obstructive pulmonary disease (COPD) exacerbation
- Pneumothorax
- Pneumonia
- Sepsis
- Acute anxiety with hyperventilation

Clinical Probability of an Acute Pulmonary Embolism

The clinical probability of PE can be assessed by including information obtained from resting electrocardiograms (ECG), chest X-ray results, patient history, PE risk factors, and physical examinations. There are several clinical prediction scores, such as the Wells score or the revised Geneva score, that may aid in the clinical assessment once we suspect the chance that there may be an acute pulmonary embolism (Yetgin at al., 2014). This is described in Tables 1 and 2. These prediction scores that are studied in patients presenting in emergency departments are composed of several clinical factors, and will help to establish the probability of PE before testing (pretest probability). For example, the Wells score result is classified as likely or unlikely for PE. Regardless of the employed model, the percent of patients with confirmed PE can be expected to be 10% in the low-probability category, 30% in the moderate-probability category, and 65% in the high probability category (Innocentin et al., 2021). When a two-level classification is used, the proportion of patients with confirmed PE is 12% in the PE-unlikely category and 30% in the PE-likely category. However, the clinical judgment of an experienced clinician might be even more sensitive, compared to results obtained from prediction scores.

PE should probably be considered more likely if one or more of the symptoms and signs, particularly dyspnea, hemoptysis, tachycardia, or hypoxemia, cannot be explained clinically, together with ECG, chest X-ray, D-dimers and urgent echocardiography results. In patients for whom the probability of PE is unlikely, only D-dimer testing in outpatients may be needed. In those patients, a negative D-dimer test (< 500 ng/l) is highly indicative of the absence of pulmonary embolism (Stein et al., 2014). However, if there is a high clinical suspicion of PE with low bleeding risk, immediate anticoagulation should be considered while the diagnosis is confirmed with additional tests.

Table 1. Modified Geneva score for pulmonary embolism probability

Variables		Points
Age>65 years		+1
Previous VTE		+3
Surgery requiring anesthesia or fracture of lower limb in the past month		+2
Active malignancy		+2
Unilateral leg pain		+3
Hemoptysis		+2
Unilateral leg edema		+4
Heart rate 75-94 bpm		+3
Heart rate >95 bpm		+5
PE probability	Score	PE prevalence
Low	=3	8%
High	>11	74%

Abbreviations: PE = pulmonary embolism, DVT= Deep vein thrombosis.

Table 2. Modified Wells criteria for pulmonary embolism probability

Features	Score points
Clinical sign and symptoms of DVT	3.0
No alternative diagnosis	3.0
Heart rate >100 beats/min	1.5
Immobilization for three days or surgery in the previous four weeks	1.5
Previous DVT or PE	1.5
Hemoptysis	1.0
Malignancy with active treatment in the past six months or under palliative care	1.0
Pretest clinical probability	
PE unlikely	=4
PE likely	>4.0

Abbreviations: PE= pulmonary embolism, DVT= Deep vein thrombosis.

One additional option for decreasing rates of testing for PE using D-dimers is the use of the PERC rule with eight criteria; however, this has similar rates of sensitivity and negative predictive values (Drescher et al., 2020). Presence of these criteria in a clinically low-risk patient implied that further testing for PE was not indicated. The PERC rule includes eight criteria: age < 50 years, heart rate < 100 bpm, oxygen saturation ≥ 95%, no prior DVT or PE, no unilateral leg swelling or hemoptysis, absence of surgery or trauma requiring hospitalization within the past four weeks, and no estrogen use.

Initial evaluation of patients with suspected PE should include pulse oximetry and chest X-rays. In addition, ECG, arterial blood gas (ABG) measurements, or both may help to exclude other diagnoses including acute coronary syndromes or pneumonia. Blood gas testing should be considered, particularly for patients with dyspnea or tachypnea who did not have hypoxemia detected with pulse oximetry (Rodger et al., 2000). Arterial or venous blood gas measurement may show an increased alveolar to arterial oxygen difference or hypocapnia. Both tests are moderately sensitive, but neither is specific for PE. We can obtain normal oxygen saturation due to a small clot burden or compensatory hyperventilation.

ECG is one of the main initial examinations in patients presenting in emergency departments with suspected PE. Most often it shows tachycardia and various ST-T wave abnormalities, which are not specific for pulmonary embolism (Figure 1). An S1Q3T3 or a new right bundle branch block (RBBB) accompanied with tachycardia may indicate the effect of a sudden rise in RV size and RV strain affecting RV conduction pathways (Shopp et al., 2015). However, these findings occur in only 5% of patients and are moderately specific, although they are more frequent in a higher percentage of patients with massive PE. Right axis deviation and P-pulmonale may be present. Atrial arrhythmias, most frequently atrial fibrillation, may also be associated with acute PE.

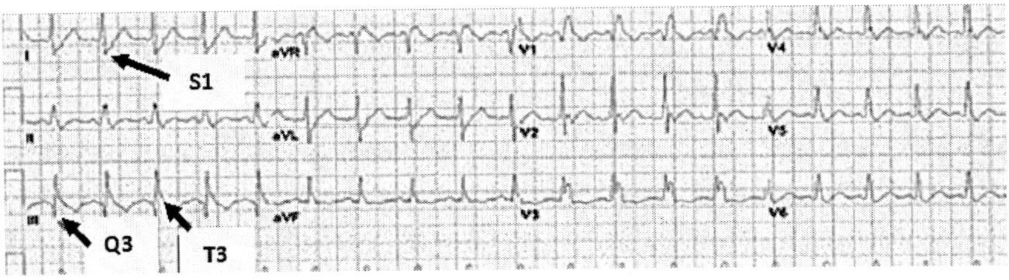

Figure 1. ECG in acute pulmonary embolism showing sinus tachycardia with heart rate 140 bpm, RBBB, and S1Q3T3 pattern.

D-Dimer Testing

Plasma D-dimer is a fibrin degradation product, and it is a marker that has been extensively studied as a diagnostic and prognostic parameter in patients with suspected and established venous thromboembolism. (Bounameaux et al., 1991). At the standardly accepted cutoff value (500 mg/L), the specificity of D-dimer for PE is low (20 to 50%), which is explained by the several conditions that activate the coagulation and fibrinolytic processes not always connected to the thromboembolic event (Righini et al., 2008). D-dimer plasma level measured with an enzyme linked immunosorbent assay (ELISA) is almost always increased in acute PE (high sensitivity -97%). Normal D-dimer plasma values exclude the disease with high certainty (negative predictive value - NPV 100%) (Taira T et al., 2010). D-dimer values below 500 mg/L used in addition to lower extremity ultrasonography in patients with low or intermediate PE clinical probability can safely rule out a PE diagnosis.

On the other hand, the positive predictive value of elevated D-dimer levels is low and D-dimer testing alone is not useful in cases with suspected PE. D-dimer is frequently elevated in several diseases, such as in patients with cancer, arterial thromboembolic disease, hospitalized patients, patients undergoing surgery and trauma, severe infection or inflammatory disease, pregnancy, heart failure, sepsis, renal and liver disease (Chopra et al., 2012). The conditions and disease that leads to increased D-dimer values are shown in Table 3. The European Society of Cardiology recommends the use of age-adjusted cutoff values of D-dimer in evaluation of patients with suspected PE. This approach may improve the performance of D-dimer testing in the elderly. A multinational prospective treatment study, which included 3346 patients, evaluated the previously validated age-adjusted cutoff (age x 10 mg/L, for patients aged >50 years) (Righini et al., 2014). The results showed a significant increase in the number of patients for whom PE can be excluded without additional false-negative findings.

Table 3. Pathological conditions and disease with elevated D-dimer values

Bleeding	Bleeding is the pathological cause of elevated D-dimer.
Thrombosis	Venous thrombosis – DVT, PE, vein thrombosis in atypical sites like upper arms, mesenteric, cerebral) Arterial thrombosis - acute coronary syndrome, stroke, peripheral artery disease, arterial thromboembolism, intestinal ischemia Microvascular thrombosis – DIC Intravascular thrombosis - catheters, pace-makers, artificial valves atrial fibrillation, LV aneurism, congestive heart failure, heart thrombus, acute aortic dissection
Cardiovascular disease	
Renal disease	
Liver disease	
Malignancy and its treatment	
Infection	Pneumonia, sepsis
Chronic inflammatory disease	
Pregnancy	Preeclampsia, HELLP Syndrome
Other	Alzheimer's disease, sickle cell disease

Abbreviations: DIC - Disseminated intravascular coagulation, LV-left ventricle, HELLP- Hemolysis, elevated liver enzymes, low platelets.

Diagnosis of Acute Pulmonary Embolism

Over the last three decades, there have been significant advances in the field of PE diagnosis, prognosis, and management, with the introduction of stepwise diagnostic strategies and simple algorithms including PE clinical probability assessment (Ortel et al., 2020). Contemporary diagnostic and management algorithms are simple, easy to use, safe, cost effective, and well standardized. These diagnostic algorithms are mainly based on the assessment of clinical pretest probability, D-dimer measurement, and imaging tests, predominantly echocardiography and computed tomography pulmonary angiography based on the patient's clinical and hemodynamic stability (Le Gal et al., 2006). Confirmatory imaging tests such as CTPA or the V/Q scan are associated with a non-negligible radiation dose and are also expensive. Therefore, current diagnostic strategies aim at identifying a group of low-risk patients, among those with suspected PE, for whom no imaging test is required. All diagnostic recommendations and proper use of imaging techniques help reduce the rate of PE misdiagnoses. Echocardiography and computer tomographic pulmonary angiography (CTPA) are the most widely used noninvasive imaging methods for PE diagnosis. However, the frequent and non-selected use of multidetector CTPA may lead to overdiagnosis and increased patient radiation exposure (Anderson et al., 2007).

Regardless of the risk stratification scoring system used, 6% of patients with confirmed PE can be expected to be in the low-probability group, 23% in the moderate-probability, and 49% in the high probability category (Ceriani et al., 2010). The reported proportion of patients with confirmed PE is 8% in the PE-unlikely category assessed by two-level classification and 34% in the PE-likely category. The diagnostic algorithms for suspected PE with and without hemodynamic instability are presented in Figures 1 and 2, respectively. However, the diagnostic approach in suspected PE patient is variable, depending on the availability and expertise in different imaging modalities in different hospital settings and health care systems. One very important point while facing the patient with suspected PE is to not miss the diagnosis that will lead to high death risk in untreated patients, or on the other hand, overtreat the patient, which may increase the bleeding risk of anticoagulant therapy.

Diagnostic Approach in Suspected PE in Patient with Hemodynamic Instability

Assessment of hemodynamic stability is critical in the initial evaluation of patients with suspected PE. Hemodynamically unstable patients, defined as massive PE, are patients who present with systolic blood pressure (BP) <90 mmHg for a period >15 minutes or a drop in systolic blood pressure substantially below baseline (generally a drop of >40 mmHg; hypotension requiring vasopressors; or clear evidence of shock with oliguria, wet and pale skin, disorientation; or patients suffering cardiac arrest with resuscitation) (Konstantinides et al., 2020). The diagnostic strategy in suspected PE with hemodynamic instability is shown in Figure 1. The clinical PE probability in this group of patients is usually high, and the differential diagnosis includes acute coronary syndrome, acute heart failure, tamponade, aortic dissection, and hypovolemia.

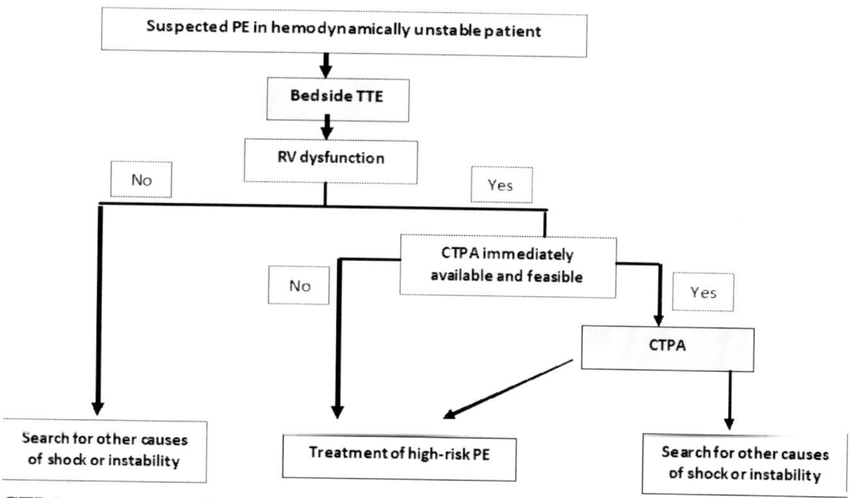

CTPA = computed tomography pulmonary angiography; CUS = compression ultrasonography; DVT = deep vein thrombosis; LV = left ventricle; PE = pulmonary embolism; RV = right ventricle; TOE = transesophageal echocardiography; TTE = transthoracic echocardiogram.

Figure 1. Diagnostic algorithm for patients with suspected high-risk pulmonary embolism and hemodynamic instability (adopted from the European Society of Cardiology guidelines on pulmonary embolism 2019) (Konstantinides et al., 2020).

The most useful initial imaging modality in patients with hemodynamic instability and high PE probability is bedside urgent echocardiography, which will show indirect signs of possible PE presence with the evidence of acute RV dysfunction as a cause of hemodynamic instability (Dronkers et al., 2017). In a critically ill patient, echocardiographic evidence of RV dysfunction with enlarged RV chambers or additional visualization of RV thrombi is sufficient to allow immediate use of reperfusion without further testing (Torbicki et al., 2004). Bedside transesophageal echocardiography may be used, which allows direct visualization of thrombi in the pulmonary artery and its main branches, especially in patients with RV dysfunction, thrombi in RV or vena cava (Casazza et al., 1997). Moreover, bedside vascular ultrasound can detect deep vein thrombosis (DVT). After hemodynamic stabilization of the patient by using evidence-based guidelines treatment, final PE diagnosis should be confirmed by CT angiography. Normal echocardiographic results, without any evidence of RV dysfunction in unstable patients, and the presence of PE as a cause of hemodynamic instability can be ruled out (Koc et al., 2016).

Diagnostic Approach in Suspected PE in Patients without Hemodynamic Instability

In hemodynamically stable patients presenting in the emergency department with suspected PE, the first diagnostic step is to assess the PE clinical probability. In cases with low and intermediate probability, the next step is to measure the plasma D-dimer using age adjusted values (Righini et al., 2004). In patients with high clinical probability, D-dimer should not be measured, because of the low NPV value in this population. D-dimer values <500 ng/l safely rule out PE with high accuracy. Performance of multidetector CTPA is the next step in patients with an elevated D-dimer level or the first step of imaging modality in patients with a high clinical PE probability (Brenner et al., 2007). Evidence of clots in the form of contrast defects, at least at the segmental level of pulmonary arteries on the CTPA, is considered to be a diagnostic finding of PE. This diagnostic approach is recommended by the latest European Society of Cardiology guidelines on the management of PE, as shown in Figure 2.

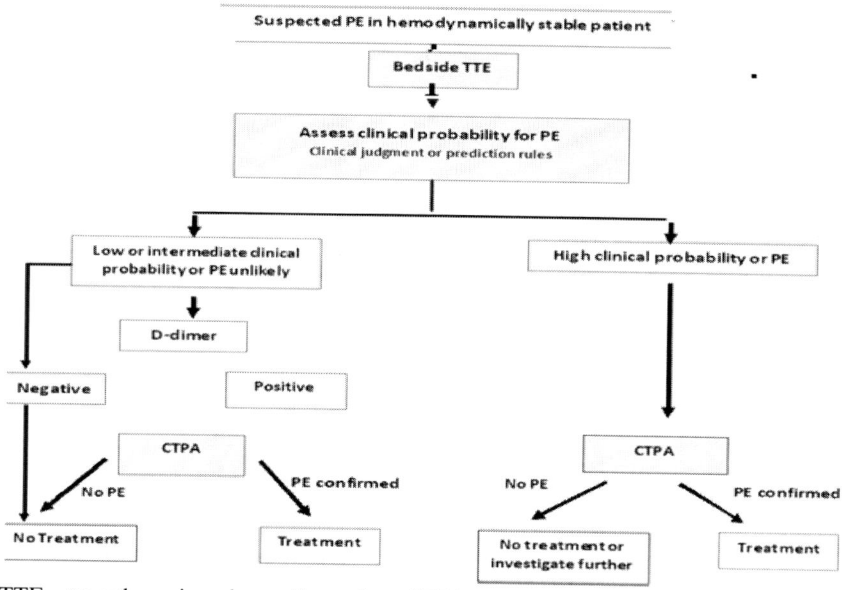

TTE= transthoracic echocardiography; CTPA = computed tomography pulmonary angiography/angiogram; PE = pulmonary embolism.

Figure 2. Diagnostic algorithm for hemodynamically stable patients with suspected pulmonary embolism (adopted from the European Society of Cardiology guidelines on pulmonary embolism 2019) (Konstantinides et al., 2020).

Overview of Current Diagnostic Strategies

Lung Scintigraphy

The clinical use of the ventilation scan is aimed to increase diagnostic specificity. In acute PE, pulmonary ventilation is expected to be normal in the hyperperfused segments (ventilation/perfusion mismatched) (Waxman et al., 2017). Ventilation-perfusion (V/Q) scans may be used for their negative predictive value; however, the results may be less reliable in patients with other conditions that may cause ventilation and perfusion mismatch such as pneumonia, atelectasis, and previous pulmonary emboli. In general, a negative V/Q scan may rule out significant pulmonary embolism (Gottschalk et al., 1993). The V/Q scan may be used in outpatients with a low clinical probability and a normal chest X-ray. It may also be used in young patients, pregnant women, patients with a history of contrast medium-induced anaphylaxis, and patients with severe renal failure, depending on local availability. This is because it is a procedure that uses low radiation and contrast medium doses. Performing only a perfusion scan might be acceptable in patients with a normal chest X-ray; any perfusion defect in this situation would be considered a mismatch. In patients with a high probability lung scan who have a low clinical probability of PE, confirmation by other tests should be considered (Bajc et al., 2008). The high frequency of non-diagnostic scans is a limitation for the use of V/Q scan, because they indicate the necessity for further diagnostic testing.

Echocardiography

Acute PE may lead to right ventricular (RV) pressure overload and dysfunction, which can be detected by echocardiography. RV has a specific geometry and morphology, and there is no individual echocardiographic parameter that provides reliable information on RV size or function. Reported negative predictive value of echocardiography for PE diagnosis is 40-50%, implying that negative results cannot reliably exclude PE (Roy et al., 2005). On the other hand, signs of RV overload or dysfunction may also be found in the absence of acute PE, and may be a result of concomitant presence of cardiorespiratory disease. Echocardiographic examination is not recommended as an initial part of the routine diagnostic approach in hemodynamically stable patients with suspected PE, although it may be useful in the differential diagnosis of acute dyspnea or chest pain (Roy et al., 2005). In patients with suspected high-risk PE, the absence of echocardiographic signs of RV overload or RV dysfunction practically excludes PE as the cause of hemodynamic instability (Grifoni et al., 2000). In the latter case, echocardiography may be of further help in the differential diagnosis of the cause of shock, by detecting pericardial tamponade, acute valvular dysfunction, severe global or regional LV dysfunction, aortic dissection, or hypovolemia. Echocardiographic presence of RV dysfunction is used for patients' risk stratification (Torbicki et al., 1999). The most common echocardiographic parameters evaluated in patients with acute PE are shown in Figure 3. The value of echocardiography in diagnosis of PE is comprehensively described in Chapter 4 of this book.

Computer Tomographic Pulmonary Angiography

In patients with suspected PE, multidetector computer tomographic pulmonary angiography (CTPA) is the gold standard for noninvasive imaging for the diagnosis or exclusion of acute PE. The method has high diagnostic accuracy, showing sensitivity and specificity of 83% and 96%, respectively, based on the Prospective Investigation on Pulmonary Embolism Diagnosis (PIOPED) II study results (Le Gal et al. 2010). The diagnosis of acute PE is based on direct evidence of a thrombus, either as a filling defect or as amputation of a pulmonary arterial branch. This technique allows visualization of a thrombus size smaller than 15 mm within the subsegmental arteries, with substantial interobserver variability at this level (Patel et al., 2003). The PIOPED II study underlines the influence of pretest clinical probability on the predictive value of multidetector CTPA. In patients with a low to intermediate clinical PE probability, a negative CTPA result had a high NPV for PE (96 and 89%, respectively); however, NPV is only 60% if the pretest probability is high. To the contrary, the positive predictive value (PPV) of a positive CTPA result is high (92-96%) in patients with an intermediate and high clinical probability, and significantly lower (58%) in patients with a low pretest likelihood of PE (Stein et al., 2006). In clinical practice, in patients with a discrepancy between clinical judgment and the CTPA result, additional testing should be considered.

Venous Ultrasonography

In the majority of patients with PE, thrombus originates from DVT in a lower limb, and rarely from an upper limb DVT, and this is primarily in patients with venous catheterization procedures. Venous ultrasonography has become the most widely used diagnostic modality for the diagnosis and exclusion of acute DVT. Compression ultrasonography (CUS) has a sensitivity of >90% and a specificity of 95% for proximal symptomatic DVT (Perrier et al., 1998). However, CUS shows a DVT only in 30-50% of patients with PE, and finding a proximal DVT in patients suspected of having PE is considered sufficient to warrant anticoagulant treatment without further testing (Kearon et al., 1998) However, patients in whom PE is indirectly confirmed by the presence of a proximal DVT should undergo risk assessment for PE severity and risk of early death. In patients admitted to the emergency department with hemodynamic instability and suspicion of PE, an echocardiogram without signs of RV dysfunction and a normal venous ultrasound can exclude PE with a high (96%) negative predictive value (Le Gal et al., 2006). When there is no evidence of lower extremity DVT and objective evidence of PE, the PE may have originated from pelvic veins or embolized completely from a lower extremity vein.

Magnetic Resonance Angiography

Magnetic resonance angiography (MRA) has been evaluated for several years regarding suspected PE (Revel et al., 2012). However, evidence from several large studies show that this modality is not yet ready for clinical practice due to its low sensitivity, its high proportion of inconclusive results, and its low availability and experience in most emergency situations. A full description of the value of imaging techniques for acute PE diagnosis is described in Chapter 4 of this book.

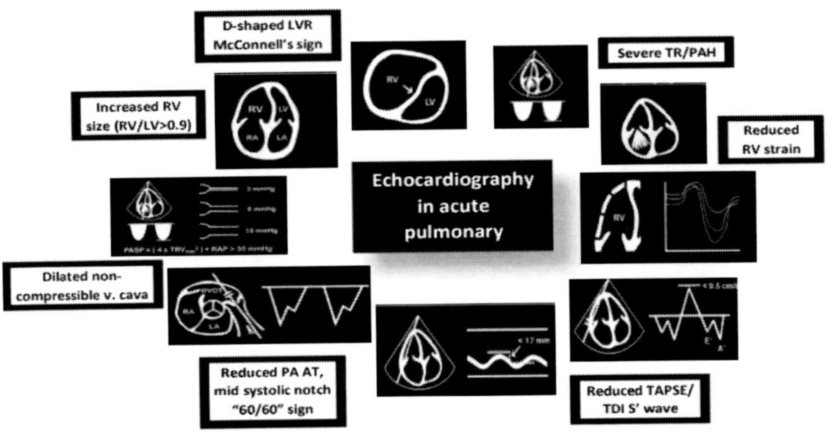

Abbreviations: RV-right ventricle, LV- left ventricle, TR- tricuspid regurgitation, PAH- pulmonary artery hypertension, PA -pulmonary artery, AT-acceleration time, TDI – tissue doppler.

Figure 3. Echocardiography parameters assessed in acute pulmonary embolism.

Conclusion

Diagnosis of pulmonary embolism is a stepwise approach necessitating high clinical suspicion, integrated use of imaging techniques and biomarkers, proper risk stratification, and individual therapy administration. The aim of all these diagnostic and risk stratification steps is reduction of PE mortality and further improvement of the patient's quality of life. Proper use of the guidelines recommending diagnostic and risk stratification algorithms, potentially leads to reduced health care costs and shortened hospitalization.

References

Anderson, D. R., Kahn, S. R., Rodger, M. A., Kovacs, M. J., Morris, T., Hirsch, A., Lang, E., Stiell, I., Kovacs, G., Dreyer, J., Dennie, C., Cartier, Y., Barnes, D., Burton, E., Pleasance, S., Skedgel, C., O'Rouke, K., Wells, P. S. Computed tomographic pulmonary angiography vs ventilation-perfusion lung scanning in patients with suspected pulmonary embolism: a randomized controlled trial. *JAMA*. 2007; 298: 27432753.

Bajc, M., Olsson, B., Palmer, J., Jonson, B. Ventilation/perfusion SPECT for diagnostics of pulmonary embolism in clinical practice. *J Intern Med*. 2008; 264: 379387.

Barco, S., Ende-Verhaar, Y. M., Becattini, C., Jimenez, D., Lankeit, M., Huisman, M. V., Konstantinides, S. V., Klok, F. A. Differential impact of syncope on the prognosis of patients with acute pulmonary embolism: a systematic review and meta-analysis. *Eur Heart J*. 2018; 39:41864195.

Bounameaux, H., Cirafici, P., De Moerloose, P., SchneiderM P. A., Slosman, D., Reber, G., Unger, P. F. Measurement of D-dimer in plasma as diagnostic aid in suspected pulmonary embolism. *Lancet*. 1991; 337: 196–200.

Brenner, D. J., Hall, E. J. Computed tomography–an increasing source of radiation exposure. *N Engl J Med*. 2007; 357: 22772284.

Burns, S. K., Haramati, L. B. Diagnostic imaging and risk stratification of patients with acute pulmonary embolism. *Cardiol Rev*. 2012 Jan-Feb; 20(1):15-24.

Casazza, F., Bongarzoni, A., Centonze, F., Morpurgo, M. Prevalence and prognostic significance of right-sided cardiac mobile thrombi in acute massive pulmonary embolism. *Am J Cardiol*. 1997; 79:1433-1435.

Ceriani, E., Combescure, C., Gal, G. L., Nendaz, M., Perneger, T., Bounameaux, H., Perrier, A., Righini, M. Clinical prediction rules for pulmonary embolism: a systematic review and meta-analysis. *J Thromb Haemost*. 2010; 8:957–970.

Chopra, N., Doddamreddy, P., Grewal, H., and Kumar, P. C. An elevated D-dimer value: a burden on our patients and hospitals. *Int J Gen Med*. 2012; 5: 87–92.

Dabbouseh, N. M., Patel, J. J., Paul Anthony Bergl. Role of echocardiography in managing acute pulmonary embolism. *Heart* 2019 Dec;105(23):1785-1792.

Drescher, M. J., Fried, J., Brass, R., Medoro, A., Murphy, T., and https://pubmed.ncbi.nlm.nih.gov/?term=Delgado J[Author] Delgado, J. Knowledge translation of the PERC rule for suspected pulmonary embolism: A blueprint for reducing the number of CT pulmonary angiograms. *West J Emerg Med.* 2017 Oct; 18(6): 1091–1097.

Dronkers, E. A., Van der Hulle. T., Le Gal. G., Kyrle, P. A., Huisman, M. V., Cannegieter, S. C., Klok, F. A. Subcommittee on predictive and diagnostic variables in thrombotic disease. Towards a tailored diagnostic standard for future diagnostic studies in pulmonary embolism: communication from the SSC of the ISTH. *J Thromb Haemost* 2017; 15:1040-1043.

Gottschalk, A., Sostman, H. D., Coleman, R. E., Juni, J. E., Thrall, J., McKusick, K. A., Froelich, J. W., Alavi, A. Ventilation-perfusion scintigraphy in the PIOPED study. Part II. Evaluation of the scintigraphic criteria and interpretations. *J Nucl Med.* 1993; 34:11191126.

Grifoni, S., Olivotto, I., Cecchini, P., Pieralli F, Camaiti, A., Santoro, G., Conti, A., Agnelli, G., Berni, G. Short-term clinical outcome of patients with acute pulmonary embolism, normal blood pressure, and echocardiographic right ventricular dysfunction. *Circ.* 2000; 101:2817-2822.

Innocentin, F., Lazzari, C., Ricci, F., Paolucci, E., Agishev, I., and Pini, R. D-dimer tests in the emergency department: current insights. *Open Access Emerg Med.* 2021; 13: 465–479.

Kearon, C., Ginsberg, J. S., Hirsh, J. The role of venous ultrasonography in the diagnosis of suspected deep venous thrombosis and pulmonary embolism. *Ann Intern Med.* 1998; 129:1044-1049.

Koc, M., Kostrubiec, M., Elikowski, W., Meneveau, N., Lankeit, M., Grifoni, S., KuchWocial, A., Petris, A., Zaborska, B., Stefanovic, B. S., Hugues, T., Torbicki, A., Konstantinides, S., Pruszczyk, P., RiHTER investigators. Outcome of patients with right heart thrombi: the Right Heart Thrombi European Registry. *Eur Respir J.* 2016; 47:869-875.

Konstantinides, S. V., Meyer, G., Becattini, C., Bueno, H., Geersing, G. J., Harjola, V. P., Huisman, M. V., Humbert, M., Jennings, C. S., Jiménez, D., Kucher, N., Lang, I. M., Lankeit, M., Lorusso, R., Mazzolai, L., Meneveau, N., Áinle, F. N., Prandoni, P., Pruszczyk, P., Righini, M., Torbicki, A., Belle, E. V., Zamorano, J. L.; ESC Scientific Document Group. ESC guidelines for the diagnosis and management of acute pulmonary embolism developed in collaboration with the European Respiratory Society (ERS). *Eur Heart J.* 2020 Jan 21;41(4):543-603.

Le Gal, G., Righini, M., Roy, P. M., Sanchez, O., Aujesky, D., Bounameaux, H., Perrier, A. Prediction of pulmonary embolism in the emergency department: the revised Geneva score. *Ann Intern Med.* 2006; 144:165171.

Le Gal, G., Righini, M., Sanchez, O., Roy, P. M., Baba-Ahmed, M., Perriers, A., Bounameaux, H. A positive compression ultrasonography of the lower limb veins is highly predictive of pulmonary embolism on computed tomography in suspected patients. *Thromb Haemost.* 2006; 95:963-966.

Le Gal, G. Subsegmental pulmonary embolism diagnosed by computed tomography: incidence and clinical implications. A systematic review and meta-analysis of the management outcome studies. *J Thromb Haemost.* 2010; 8:1716-1722.

Miniati, M., Prediletto, R., Formichi, B., Marini, C., Di Ricco, G., Tonelli, L., Allescia, G., Pistolesi, M. Accuracy of clinical assessment in the diagnosis of pulmonary embolism. *Am J Respir Crit Care Med.* 1999;159:864-871.

Ortel, T. L., Neumann, I., Ageno, W., Beyth, R., Clark, N. P., Cuker, A., Hutten, B. A., Jaff, M. R., Manja, V., Schulman, S., Thurston, C., Vedantham, S., Verhamme, P., Witt, D. M., Florez, I. D., Izcovich, A., Nieuwlaat, R., Ross, S., Schünemann, H. J., Wiercioch. W., Zhang, Y., Zhang, Y. American Society of Hematology 2020 guidelines for management of venous thromboembolism: treatment of deep vein thrombosis and pulmonary embolism. *Blood Adv*. 2020 Oct 13; 4(19): 4693-4738.

Patel, S., Kazerooni, E. A., Cascade, P. N. Pulmonary embolism: optimization of small pulmonary artery visualization at multi-detector row CT. *Radiology.* 2003; 227:455-460.

Perrier, A., Bounameaux, H. Ultrasonography of leg veins in patients suspected of having pulmonary embolism. *Ann Intern Med.*1998; 128:243-243.

Pollack, C. V., Schreiber, D., Goldhaber, S. Z., Slattery, D., Fanikos, J., O'Neil, B. J., Thompson, J. R., Hiestand, B., Briese, B. A., Pendleton, R. C., Miller, C. D., Kline, J. A. Clinical characteristics, management, and outcomes of patients diagnosed with acute pulmonary embolism in the emergency department: initial report of EMPEROR (Multicenter Emergency Medicine Pulmonary Embolism in the Real World Registry). *J Am Coll Cardiol.* 2011;57:700-706.

Revel, M. P., Sanchez, O., Couchon, S., Planquette, B., Hernigou, A., Niarra, R., Meyer, G., Chatellier, G. Diagnostic accuracy of magnetic resonance imaging for an acute pulmonary embolism: results of the 'IRM-EP' study. *J Thromb Haemost.* 2012; 10:743750.

Righini, M., Aujesky, D., Roy, P. M., Cornuz, J., De Moerloose, P., Bounameaux, H., Perrier, A. Clinical usefulness of D-dimer depending on clinical probability and cutoff value in outpatients with suspected pulmonary embolism. *Arch Intern Med. 2004*; 164:24832487.

Righini, M., Perrier, A., De Moerloose, P., Bounameaux, H. D-dimer for venous thromboembolism diagnosis: 20 years later. *J Thromb Haemost*. 2008; 6:1059–71.

Righini, M., Robert-Ebadi, H., Le Gal, G. Diagnosis of acute pulmonary embolism. *J Thromb Haemost.* 2017;15:12511261.

Righini, M., Van Es, J., Den Exter, P. L., Roy, P. M., Verschuren, F., Ghuysen, A., Rutschmann, O. T., Sanchez, O., Jaffrelot, M., Trinh-Duc, A., Le Gall, C., Moustafa, F., Principe, A., Van Houten, A., Ten Wolde, M., Douma, R. A., Hazelaar, G., Erkens, P. M., Van Kralingen, K. W., Grootenboers, M. J., Durian, M. F., Cheung, Y. W., Meyer, G., Bounameaux, H., Huisman, M. V., Kamphuisen, P. W., Le Gal, P. G. Age-adjusted D-dimer cutoff levels to rule out pulmonary embolism: the ADJUST-PE study. *JAMA.* 2014; 311:11171124.

Rodger, M. A., Carrier, M., Jones, G. N., Rasuli, P., Raymond, F., Djunaedi, H., Wells, P. S. Diagnostic value of arterial blood gas measurement in suspected pulmonary embolism. *Am J Respir Crit Care Med.* 2000; 162:2105-2108.

Rodríguez-Núñez, N., Ruano-Raviña, A., Lama, A., Ferreiro, L., Ricoy, J., Álvarez-Dobaño, J. M., Antelo, J. S., Toubes, M. E., Rábade, C., Golpe, A., Lourido, T., González-Barcala, J. F. and Valdés, L. Impact of cardiovascular risk factors on the clinical presentation and survival of pulmonary embolism without identifiable risk factor. *J Thorac Dis.* 2020 Oct;12(10):5411-5419.

Roy, P. M., Colombet, I., Durieux, P., Chatellier, G., Sors, H., Meyer, G. Systematic review and meta-analysis of strategies for the diagnosis of suspected pulmonary embolism. *BMJ.* 2005; 331:259.

Shopp, J. D., Stewart, L. K., Emmett, T. W., Kline, J. A. Findings from 12-lead electrocardiography that predict circulatory shock from pulmonary embolism: systematic review and meta-analysis. *Acad Emerg Med.* 2015; 22:1127-1137.

Stein, P. D., Fowler, S. E., Goodman, L. R., Gottschalk, A., Hales, C. A., Hull, R. D., Leeper, K. V., Popovich, J., Quinn, D. A., Sos, T. A., Sostman, H. D., Tapson, V. F., Wakefield, T. W., Weg J. G., Woodard P. K.; PIOPED II investigators. Multidetector computed tomography for acute pulmonary embolism. *N Engl J Med.* 2006;354: 2317-2327.

Stein, P. D., Hull, R. D., Patel, K. C., Olson, R. E., Ghali, W. A., Brant, R., Biel, R. K., Bharadia, V., Kalra, N. K. D-dimer for the exclusion of acute venous thrombosis and pulmonary embolism: A systematic review. *Ann Intern Med.* 2004; 140:589–602.

Taira, T., Taira, B. R., Carmen, M., Chohan, J., Singer, A. J. Risk of venous thromboembolism in patients with borderline quantitative D-dimer levels. *Am J Emerg Med.* 2010; 28:450–3.

Torbicki, A., Galie,´N., Covezzoli, A., Rossi, E., De Rosa, M., Goldhaber, S. Z.; ICOPER Study Group. Right heart thrombi in pulmonary embolism: results from the International Cooperative Pulmonary Embolism Registry. *J Am Coll Cardiol.* 2003; 41:22452251.

Torbicki, A., Kurzyna, M, Ciurzynski, M., Pruszczyk, P., Pacho, R., Kuch-Wocial, A., Szulc, M., Proximal pulmonary emboli modify right ventricular ejection pattern. *Eur Respir J.* 1999; 13:616-621.

Waxman, A. D., Bajc, M., Brown, M., Fahey, F. H., Freeman, L. M., Haramati, L. B., Julien, P., Le Gal, G., Neilly, B., Rabin, J., Soudry, G., Tapson, V., Torbati, S., Kauffman, J., Ahuja, S., Donohoe, K. Appropriate use criteria for ventilation-perfusion imaging in pulmonary embolism: summary and excerpts. *J Nucl Med.* 2017; 58:13N15N. 118.

Yetgin, G. O., Aydin, S. A., Koksal, O., Ozdemir, F., Mert, D. K., Gokhan, Torun, G. Clinical probability and risk analysis of patients with suspected pulmonary embolism. *World J Emerg Med.* 2014; 5(4): 264–269.

Chapter 3

Risk Stratification and an Assessment of Pulmonary Embolism Severity

Irena Mitevska*, PhD
University Cardiology Clinic, Clinical Center, Medical Faculty, Saints Cyril and Metodij University, Skopje, North Macedonia

Abstract

Pulmonary embolism (PE) is a serious condition whose mortality and prognosis depends on a fast diagnosis, PE causes, the patient's clinical presentation, as well as comorbidities and hemodynamic repercussions of the acute pulmonary artery thrombosis. Risk stratification of patients with acute PE is mandatory for appropriate management decisions. Initial risk stratification is based on clinical symptoms and signs of hemodynamic instability, which indicate a high risk of early death. In the large remaining group of patients with PE who are hemodynamically stable, further risk stratification requires the assessment of additional prognostic criteria: clinical, imaging, and laboratory indicators of the PE severity, which are not only related to the presence of RV dysfunction but also to the presence of comorbidities that may have a negative influence on early prognosis. On the other hand, low-risk patients are candidates for early discharge and home treatment and have a better prognosis. Treatment based on appropriate individual risk stratification determines the patient's outcome, length and cost of hospitalization, and our actions in case of sudden clinical deterioration.

Keywords: risk stratification, risk scores, prognosis, imaging

* Corresponding Author's Email: peovksai@yahoo.com.

In: Pulmonary Embolism
Editors: Irena Mitevska, Sonja Salinger, Marijan Bosevski et al.
ISBN: 979-8-89113-175-0

Introduction

Pulmonary embolism patients may have a wide spectrum of clinical presentation, ranging from asymptomatic to life-threatening PE presenting with cardiogenic shock. Risk stratification is one of the most basic and critical points in the management of acute PE, which guides both diagnostic and treatment approaches. An estimated 10% of patients with pulmonary embolisms die within the first few hours after presentation (Bělohlávek et al., 2013). It is assumed that around 5% of PE patients are high risk, 45% have intermediate-risk and an additional 50% are low-risk patients. Many patients with acute PE die before hospitalization without diagnosis confirmation (Morrone et al., 2018). In most of these patients, PE is not suspected as a possible diagnosis. Depending on the assessed individual risk, treatment with thrombolysis or embolectomy may be indicated in high-risk patients. To the contrary, early hospital discharge or anticoagulation home treatment may be considered in low-risk PE patients. The most challenging group are the intermediate-high-risk patients, since they have an increased risk of adverse outcomes. They might benefit from a more aggressive approach, including rescue reperfusion therapy, reduced intravenous or catheter thrombolysis, and more intensive monitoring. The contemporary approach that includes a combination of markers of the right ventricular dysfunction and myocardial injury, has an insufficient positive predictive value to guide primary thrombolysis (Konstantinides et al., 2020). Additional markers such as plasma lactate, which are more sensitive parameters of circulatory failure, have shown good prognostic accuracy and have an important role in individual risk stratification and prognosis. The approach for reducing PE mortality includes an increase of the clinical suspicion level of PEs, shortening the time needed for diagnosis and initiation of anticoagulation therapy, risk-stratification improvement, and using appropriate thromboprophylaxis in selected at-risk patients.

Classification of Risk

The outcome of the patients with acute PE most directly correlates with the degree of PE hemodynamic repercussion and presence of RV dysfunction. The latest European Society of Cardiology guidelines on pulmonary embolism recommend an individual risk stratification of early PE-related death

(Konstantinides et al., 2020). Based on the presence or absence of abnormal values of these parameters, patients are divided into four risk groups: high-risk patients, intermediate-high-risk, intermediate-low-risk, and low-risk patients, as shown in Table 1. High-risk PE patients have intrahospital or 30-day mortality risk of over 15% and intrahospital mortality in patients with shock is reported to be around 56%. Intermediate-high-risk patients are a heterogenous population additionally stratified into intermediate-high- and intermediate-low-risk (with short-term mortality risk of 3 to 15%) (Ergan et al., 2016). The final group comprises patients with low-risk (short-term mortality risk of less than 1%).

Clinical Parameters of Pulmonary Embolism Severity

Hemodynamic instability is defined based on the following parameters: presence of obstructive shock with systolic blood pressure (SBP) <90 mmHg, need of vasopressor support, presence of pale and wet peripheral skin, oliguria, signs of end-organ hypoperfusion, or SBP below 90 mmHg for more than 15 min in the absence of hypovolemia, sepsis or arrhythmia or resuscitated cardiac arrest (Konstantinides et al., 2020). Several additional parameters including tachycardia, hypotension, respiratory insufficiency with tachypnea and low oxygen saturation, syncope, alone or in combination. These have also have been associated with a worsened short-term prognosis in acute PE. Presence of imaging parameters of right ventricular (RV) dysfunction, thrombus location and CT angiographic markers of PE extensity as well as increased plasma biomarkers are an essential part of the assessment of PE severity (Torbicki et al., 2003).

Biomarkers in the Assessment of Pulmonary Embolism Risk

Markers of Right Ventricular Dysfunction

Cardiac Troponin

In patients with acute PE, troponin values are increased due to the presence of RV dysfunction, increased pressures, and stretching of the RV myocardium, with further increases in the cases of progression to the state of shock (Barco et al., 2019). Assessment of high sensitive troponin values are an essential part of the patient's risk stratification. Cardiac troponin elevation is defined as concentrations above the normal limits, which thresholds depending on the assay used. The prognostic value of troponins was evaluated in a meta-analysis on 1985 patients (Becattini et al., 2007). Elevated troponin was associated with increased short-term mortality in the total patient population and in the subgroup of stable normotensive patients (OR 5.90, 95% CI 2.68 to 12.95, with overall short-term mortality of 17.9% (Aksay et al., 2007). Another meta-analysis showed that elevated troponin concentrations were associated with an increased risk of mortality, both in unselected patients (OR 5.2, 95% CI 3.38.4) and in those who were hemodynamically stable at presentation (OR 5.9, 95% CI 2.713.0).195 The values of troponins should be evaluated in combination with other prognostic factors (Bajaj et al., 2015, Jiménez et al., 2015). Increased cardiac troponins values have relatively low specificity and positive predictive value for early mortality in normotensive patients. On the opposite side of the spectrum, acute PE risk stratification, high sensitivity troponin values have a high negative predictive value.

Brain Natriuretic Peptides

RV pressure or volume overload due to acute PE is associated with increased myocardial stretch, which leads to the release of B-type natriuretic peptide (BNP) and N-terminal (NT)-proBNP. Blood levels of natriuretic peptides reflect the severity of RV dysfunction and hemodynamic compromise in acute PE. Results from meta-analysis found that 51% of 1132 unselected patients with acute PE had elevated BNP or NT-proBNP concentrations on admission; these patients had a 10% risk of early death (95% CI 8.013%) and a 23% (95% CI 2026%) risk of an adverse clinical outcome (Lega et al., 2009). Elevated BNP or NT-proBNP concentrations similarly to the high-sensitive troponin I have low specificity and positive predictive value for early mortality in stable normotensive patients with PE; however, low NT-proBNP values worsened early in hospital outcome, with high sensitivity and a negative predictive value. It is recommended to use an NT-proBNP cutoff value >600 pg/mL for individual prognostic assessment (Lankeit et al., 2014). A meta-analysis of five recent studies reported a relative risk for the complicated clinical course of 5.63 (95% CI 2.77 to 11.43) in patients with NT-proBNP values over 1000 pg/mL (Nithianandan et al., 2020). Other validated biomarkers, which have been less extensively studied, such as heart fatty acid-binding protein, serum creatinine and copeptin, are not routinely available in daily clinical practice in many centers (Hellenkamp et al., 2015, Chopard et al., 2021, Dellas et al., 2010).

Table 1. Pulmonary embolism severity classification and risk of early intrahospital or 30-day death risk. Adopted from the European Society of Cardiology Pulmonary Embolism guidelines (Konstantinides et al., 2020)

Early mortality risk		Parameters of risk			
		Hemodynamic instability	Clinical parameters of PE severity and/or comorbidity: PESI class III-V or sPESI≥1	RV dysfunction on TTE or CTPA	Elevated cardiac troponin levels
High		+	+	+	+
Intermediate	Intermediate-high	-	+	+	+
	Intermediate-low	-	+	One or none positive	
Low		-	-	-	Assessment optional, if assessed negatively

Abbreviations: RV- right ventricle; TTE- transesophageal echocardiography; CTPA- computed tomography pulmonary angiography.

Lactates

Blood lactate level is another biomarker presenting an imbalance between tissue oxygen supply and demand, which is a result of severe PE with advanced hemodynamic instability. Elevated arterial plasma levels over 2 mmol/L predict PE-related complications, both in stable and high-risk PE patients (Konstantinides et al., 2020). A retrospective study including 287 patients with acute PE reported a significant association between plasma lactate levels above 2 mmol/L and in-hospital and 30-day mortality (OR 4.6; 95% CI 1.57 to 13.53), independent of the hemodynamic state, hypotension, right ventricular dysfunction or elevated troponin values (Vanni et al., 2011). A registry of 419 PE patients reported that lactate levels above 3.3 mmol/L had the best predictive performance for in-hospital adverse events (PPV 0.27 and NPV 0.97) (Ebner et al., 2021). Intermediate-high-risk patients with venous lactate ≥3.3 mmol/L had a 27.5% prevalence of adverse events, versus 6.8% if lactate was <3.3 mmol/L, with low-risk in the same patient's group with lactate levels <2.3 mmol/L (Ebner et al., 2021). Elevated serum creatinine levels and cystatin C values, reduced renal function, and hyponatremia are related to short-term 30-day all-cause mortality in acute PE. Vasopressin, which is released in patients with hypotension, low cardiac output, and shock and copeptin, have also been reported as useful bio parameters for risk stratification of patients with acute PE.

Noninvasive Imaging Modalities in Diagnosis of Acute Pulmonary Embolism

Acute RV failure, defined as a progressive clinical syndrome with congestion caused by impaired RV filling and/or reduced RV output, is a critical determinant of the intrahospital outcome in acute PE. Focused bedside echocardiography is an essential method for assessment of RV function in acute PE patients. It is indicated in patients with high PE probability as an initial examination, as well as during hospitalization in intermediate-risk patients in order to further risk stratify them. The role of noninvasive imaging modalities including echocardiography, CT pulmonary angiography, ventilation perfusion scan, and magnetic resonance in the diagnosis and prognosis of pulmonary embolism are described in Chapter 4.

Clinical Risk Scores

The main consequences of a PE episode are hemodynamic. Large and multiple emboli might abruptly increase pulmonary vascular resistance to a level of afterload, which cannot be matched by the right ventricle (RV), and sudden death may occur. In the ICOPER registry, the 14-day mortality of APE was above 20% (Goldhaber et al., 1999). In the RIETE registry, at three months, the cumulative rates of overall mortality and fatal PE were 8.65% and 1.68%, respectively (Jimenez et al., 2010). In the EMPEROR registry, the all-cause 30-day mortality rate was 5.4% (95% CI: 4.4% to 6.6%) (Pollack et al., 2019). Acute PE has become one of the leading causes of preventable hospital deaths. In addition to the clinical, imaging, and laboratory findings, which are directly linked to PE severity and PE-related early death, additional parameters related to the worsening conditions and comorbidity are necessary to assess a patient's overall mortality risk and early outcome. One of the most extensively validated clinical scores integrating PE severity and comorbidity is the Pulmonary Embolism Severity Index (PESI), which score points as shown in Table 2. PESI and the simplified PESI score (sPESI) have lower specificity to predict early intrahospital mortality (Dunn et al., 2012).

The drawback of these scores is their strong reliance on demographic data and comorbidities, and then on the severity of the acute PE event. PESI has discriminative power to predict the short-term death and adverse outcome events in patients with acute PE. Both scores have similar accuracy, while sPESI is easier to use (Laporte et al., 2008). A meta-analysis of 21 studies showed a significant association of low-risk PESI with lower all-cause mortality (OR 0.13; 95% CI 0.12 to 0.15), PE-related mortality (OR 0.09; 95% CI 0.05 to 0.17), and serious adverse events (OR 0.34; 95% CI 0.29 to 0.41), with no homogeneity across studies (Xiao-Yu Zhou et al., 2021). The simplified PESI includes six variables (age over 80 years, history of cancer, history of chronic cardiorespiratory disease, heart rate, systolic blood pressure, and oxygen saturation. Patients with none of the variables (0 points) are categorized as low-risk for 30 days mortality (1.1%). Patients with one to six variables (1-6 points) are categorized as high-risk with 30 days mortality risk (8.9%) (Konstantinides et al., 2020). Clinical scores alone are inadequate to guide admission to intensive care units or to initiate reperfusion therapies.

Table 2. Simplified Pulmonary Embolism Severity Index (sPESI)

sPESI score	
Variable	Points
Age > 80 y	1
History of cancer	1
History of chronic cardiopulmonary disease	1
Pulse > 110 beats/min	1
Systolic blood pressure <100 mmHg	1
Arterial oxyhemoglobin saturation (SaO2) <90%	1

Note: A total points score for individual patient is obtained by totaling the points. Risk score low – point 0; Risk score high- point >1.

Table 3. Bova Score for risk assesment in acute pulmonary embolism

Bova score	
Variable	Points
Systolic blood pressure 90-100 mmHg	2
Cardiac troponin elevation	2
Right ventricular dysfunction (Echocardiography or CT scan)	2
Pulse > 110 beats/min	1

Abbreviations: CT- computed tomography The total point score is produced by the sum of variable points (Bova risk score range: 0-7). Bova risk staging in increased with the value of total point score: stage I (0-2 points); stage II (2-4 points); stage III (>4 points).

Another score stratifying the 30-day mortality risk, is the Bova score, which was obtained from pooled results of six prospective studies on 2874 patients with stable acute PE. This score has seven-points comprising four clinical variables: heart rate ≥ 110 beats/min (1 point), systolic blood pressure 90–100 mm Hg (2 points), right ventricular dysfunction (2 points), and elevated cardiac troponin (2 points) (Bova et al., 2014), as shown in Table 3. The Bova score categorizes normotensive PE patients into three stages: risk class I (0–2 points), class II (3–4 points) and class III (>4 points), with 30-day PE related adverse events rates of 4.2%, 10.8%, and 29.2%. Several studies have shown that the risk class assessed by the Bova score significantly correlated with short-term PE- related complications and mortality. The cumulative incidence of 30 day PE-related death was 3.8% for stage I, 10.8% for stage II and 19.9% for stage III (1.9, 5.5 and 12.1 for 30-day PE mortality) with an AUC of 0.73 (Fernandez et al., 2015).

High-Risk Patients with Acute Pulmonary Embolism

Identification of high-risk patients based on the presence of hemodynamic instability is recommended for fast initiation of reperfusion therapy, since those patients have the highest mortality risk (Konstantinides et al., 2020).

The most frequent complication of acute PE is right ventricular dysfunction, which can lead to a state of circulatory shock and death. Patients with signs of hemodynamic instability are considered high-risk according to the latest ESC criteria. Data from a systematic review including 40,000 patients with PE reported short-term mortality of 19% among unstable PE patients compared to 5.7% among patients with stable PE (OR 5.9; 95% CI 2.7 to 13.0) (Leidi et al., 2022). In a study with 7438 Chinese patients, the prevalence of unstable PE was 4.2% with a mortality rate of 15.8% (Zhai et al., 2021). It is important to emphasize that the presence of hypotension alone does not define high patient risk; rather, systolic blood pressure should be considered as a continuous risk marker in patient risk assessment (Quezada et al., 2019). In the latest ESC PE guidelines from 2019 recommendations, high patient risk has been enriched by additional variables, such as evidence of end-organ dysfunction and exclusion of alternative causes of shock (Konstantinides et al., 2020, Silvy et al., 2008). Analysis of several clinical, imaging, and biomarker parameters is indicated for better prognostic assessment. Incorporation of CT angiographic PE thrombus extensity, clinical presentation, and sudden deterioration, acute renal failure, presence of proximal DVT, increased high-sensitive Troponin I. NT-proBNP, lactate values >2, and presence of RV dysfunction may identify intermediate-high-risk patient with the increased risk of clinical worsening and need of intravenous or catheter fibrinolytic therapy based on the patient's bleeding risk (Aaron et al., 2014).

Intermediate-Risk Patients with Acute Pulmonary Embolism

Approximately 45% of patients with acute pulmonary embolisms are categorized as intermediate-risk with an overall 30-day mortality between 5% and 15% (Aujesky et al., 2005. This group of patients is highly heterogeneous, with the vast majority experiencing a favorable outcome with anticoagulant therapy alone, and a small, percent of patients requiring rescue reperfusion treatment and cardiopulmonary resuscitation. Based on these facts, in the last decades efforts have been made to identify a subgroup of patients at risk of deterioration who might benefit from initial aggressive therapy and admission to intensive care units. Intermediate-risk patients are a heterogeneous group further divided into intermediate-high- and intermediate-low-risk groups. Current guidelines recommend admission of intermediate–high-risk patients to monitored intensive care unit for early detection of clinical deterioration and the potential need for rescue reperfusion. Clinically stable patients with sPESI score >1, presence of RV dysfunction, and increased hs-Troponin I values are classified as intermediate-high-risk patients. Stable patients who do not have RV dysfunction or increased hs-Troponin I values or have only one of them increased are classified as intermediate-low-risk patients (Konstantinides et al., 2020). This group has lower intrahospital and 30-day complication risks and can be treated on the ward units. In a prospective study with 1015 consecutive hemodynamically stable patients with acute PE, all causes of 30-day mortality were significantly higher in intermediate–high-risk patients (10%) than in those with low-risk or intermediate-low-risk (4%) (Mirambeaux, et al., 2019).

Data on early mortality in hemodynamically stable intermediate-risk patients from seven studies that included 1597 patients revealed an OR of 4.19 (95% CI 1.3912.58) for death from any cause in the presence of RV dysfunction with comparable magnitude of risk for elevated cardiac troponin levels (El-Menyar et al., 2019). Early all-cause mortality rates were 1.8% for RV dysfunction and 3.8% for elevated troponin levels, both in the lower range of those results reported for intermediate-risk PE. Patients with an sPESI score of 0 and signs of RV dysfunction or elevated cardiac biomarkers, should be classified and treated as intermediate-low-risk category.

Clinical Importance of Improved Identification of Intermediate-High-Risk Patients

Recommended risk prediction models and scores, including markers of circulatory dysfunction, enable us to identify a subgroup of patients with a significantly increased risk of adverse events who might potentially benefit from more aggressive therapy. The most clinically challenging group include intermediate-high-risk patients who can potentially deteriorate rapidly during the first 24-72 hours period of intensive care treatment. An example is the combination of the basal risk observed in the PEITHO trial and the positive likelihood ratio of elevated blood lactates in the sophistication of the risk (Vanni et al., 2013). The absence of hemodynamic collapse or persistent hypotension at presentation is generally thought to predict a favorable early outcome, provided that the disease is diagnosed correctly and anticoagulation is started without delay (Grifoni et al., 2000). However, some of the (initially) normotensive patients with acute PE may have an elevated risk of death or major complications (intermediate-risk PE in Europe; sub-massive PE in North America), which warrants further risk stratification and possibly specific advanced therapy.

Low-Risk Patients and Criteria for Early Discharge

Early Hospital Discharge and Outpatient Management of Low-Risk Pulmonary Embolism

Risk stratification of patients with acute PE and short-term mortality prediction rules have been developed in order to identify patients at a low-risk of mortality who could be treated as outpatients or are candidates for early hospital discharge within 48 hours. Patients with an sPESI score of 0, without the presence of RV dysfunction or increased cardiac biomarkers (hs-Troponin I) are categorized as low-risk for early mortality and are candidates for early discharge and home treatment. A study evaluating 344 low-risk PE patients randomly allocated to outpatient versus inpatient management, showed that

90-day mortality was non-inferior in outpatients compared to patients admitted in-hospital (0.6% in both groups, upper confidence limit (UCL) for difference 2.1%), scored similar results for PE recurrence (0.6% in outpatients versus 0% for inpatients, UCL 2.7%) (Aujesky et al., 2011). When evaluating patients who are potential candidates for early discharge, three criteria need to be met before assessing home treatment of a patient with acute PE: (1) low-risk of early PE-related serious complications that would require a prolonged hospital stay; (2) absence of serious comorbidity or chronic worsened diseases; and (3) the certainty and present conditions of proper outpatient care and anticoagulant treatment, taking into account the patient's compliance, family and social support, as well as the local infrastructure enabling fast access to medical care (Aujesky et al., 2011).

The sPESI score is the most frequently used tool for risk stratification of acute PE. However, this score was not developed as a selection tool for home treatment of patients, and therefore, it should be combined with additional criteria. The introduction of Hestia exclusion criteria, which represents a checklist of clinical parameters and questions that integrate comorbidities, PE severity, and feasibility conditions of home treatment enable us to more properly select low-risk patients who can be early discharged and treated at home. If the answer to one or more of the questions is "yes," the patient cannot be a candidate for early discharge. Hestia criteria are shown in Table 4. Further research should involve patients over age 80 and cancer patients who are not part of the Hestia criteria (Zondag et al., 2011).

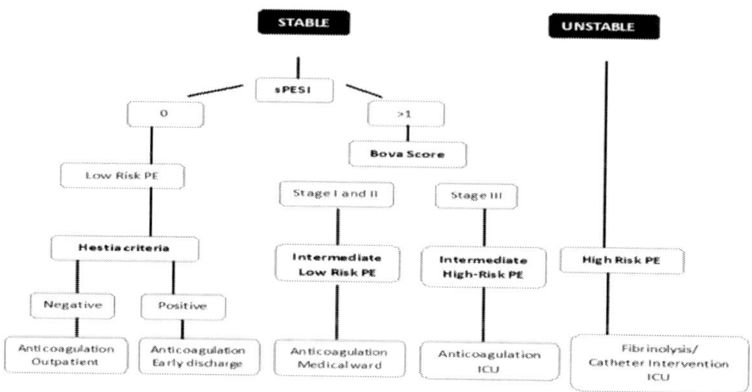

Abbreviations: ICU- intensive care unit.

Figure 1. Stepwise approach to acute pulmonary embolism risk stratification using risk scores.

Table 4. Hestia criteria for early discharge of patients with acute pulmonary embolism

Hestia Criteria	
1.	Hemodynamically unstable?
2.	Thrombolysis or embolectomy necessary?
3.	Active bleeding or high risk of bleeding?
4.	Oxygen supply to maintain oxygen >90% >24 hours?
5.	Pulmonary embolism diagnosed during anticoagulant treatment?
6.	Intravenous pain medication >24 hours?
7.	Medical or social reason for treatment in hospital >24 hours?
8.	Creatinine clearance less than 30 ml/min?
9.	Severe liver impairment?
10.	Pregnant?
11.	Documented history of heparin-induced thrombocytopenia?
-	If any of the above are answered "yes," the patient should NOT be treated as outpatient
-	An answer of "no" to all of the above meets the criteria for outpatient therapy.

In a single-arm management trial that used these criteria to select candidates for home treatment, the three-month rate of recurrent VTE was 2.0% (0.8-4.3%) in patients with acute PE who were discharged within 24 hours (Frederikus et al., 2020). Currently available scientific and clinical data indicate that both the Hestia rule and sPESI score appear to be appropriate and reliable for identifying patients who are at low PE-related risk in the absence of serious comorbidity. Both scores may be used in clinical practice according to local experience and preference. Integration and practical use of all the abovementioned risk scores for clinical approach in patients with acute PE are shown in Figure 1.

Integration of Concomitant Comorbidities into Risk Assessment of Acute Pulmonary Embolism

Clinical outcome of patients with acute PE additionally depends on the presence of comorbidities, concomitant proximal deep vein thrombosis (DVT), and bleeding complications. In a meta-analysis investigating 8859 patients with PE, the presence of concomitant DVT was confirmed as a predictor of 30-day all-cause mortality (OR 1.9, 95% CI 1.52.4), although it did not predict PE-related adverse outcomes at 90 days (Barca-Hernando et al., 2020). The outcome in patients with chronic cardiopulmonary disease, advanced age, infections, gastrointestinal disease, acute renal failure or active cancer is worse when compared to patients not having those comorbidities.

Concurrent cancer diagnosis in patients hospitalized for acute PE was associated with a 90% increase in all-cause mortality, longer length of stay, higher total charges for hospitalization, and higher rates of home health services upon discharge.

Conclusion

Treatment and prognosis of patients with acute PE requires fast, accurate stepwise risk stratification. Several risk prediction models, which include clinical variables, noninvasive imaging parameters, RV functions, and biomarkers have been developed to identify the subgroup of patients with a significant risk of early adverse events who might benefit from more aggressive treatment. Hemodynamic instability identifies high-risk patients who have the worst prognosis and are candidates for thrombolysis or catheter-directed reperfusion techniques. Clinical scores, such as sPESI, Bova, and Hestia scores, allow us to identify intermediate-high- and low-risk patients who should be treated in intensive care units or can be safely treated as outpatients. The intermediate-risk group is highly heterogeneous and the most challenging group of patients, with favorable short-term prognosis for most of them. Adherence and use of the recommended risk scores enable us to properly treat patients with acute PE and improves the prognosis of this potentially lethal condition.

References

Aksay, E., Yanturali, S., Kiyan, S. Can elevated troponin I levels predict complicated clinical course and inhospital mortality in patients with acute pulmonary embolism? *Am J Emerg Med.* 2007 Feb; 25(2):138-43.

Andersson, T., Söderberg, S. Incidence of acute pulmonary embolism, related comorbidities and survival; analysis of a Swedish national cohort. *BMC Cardiovasc Disord.* 2017; 17: 155.

Aujesky, D., Obrosky, D. S, Stone, R. A., Auble, T. E., Perrier, A., Cornuz, J., Roy, P. M., Fine, M. J. Derivation and validation of a prognostic model for pulmonary embolism. *Am J Respir Crit Care Med.* 2005; 172:1041–1046.

Aujesky, D., Roy, P. M., Verschuren, F., Righini, M., Osterwalder, J., Egloff, M., Renaud, B., Verhamme, P., Stone, R. A., Legall, C., Sanchez, O., Pugh, N. A., N'gako, A., Cornuz, J., Hugli, O., Beer, H. J., Perrier, A., Fine, M. J, Yealy D. M. Outpatient versus inpatient treatment for patients with acute pulmonary embolism: an international, open-label, randomised, non-inferiority trial. *Lancet.* 2011; 378 (9785):41–48.

Bajaj, A., Saleeb, M., Rathor, P., Sehgal, V., Kabak, B., Hosur, S. Prognostic value of troponins in acute nonmassive pulmonary embolism: a meta-analysis. *Heart Lung.* 2015; 44:327–334.

Barca-Hernando, M., Ortega-Rivera, R., Lopez-Ruz, S., Elias-Hernandez, T., Isabel Asensio-Cruz. M., Marin-Romero, S, Toral, J., Montero, E., Sanchez, V., Arellano, E., Sanchez-Diaz J. M., Real-Dominguez M., Otero-Candelera, R., and Jara-Palomares, L. Prognostic significance of incidental deep vein thrombosis in patients with cancer presenting with incidental pulmonary embolism. *Cancers* (Basel). 2020 Aug; 12(8): 2267.

Barco, S., Mahmoudpour, S. H., Planquette, B., Sanchez, O., Konstantinides, S. V., Meyer, G. Prognostic value of right ventricular dysfunction or elevated cardiac biomarkers in patients with low-risk pulmonary embolism: a systematic review and meta-analysis. *Eur Heart J* 2019; 40:902–910.

Becattini, C., Vedovati, M. C., Agnelli, G. Prognostic value of troponins in acute pulmonary embolism: a meta-analysis. *Circ.* 2007; 116:427–433.

Bělohlávek, J., Dytrych, V., Linhart, A. Pulmonary embolism, part I: epidemiology, risk factors and risk stratification, pathophysiology, clinical presentation, diagnosis and nonthrombotic pulmonary embolism. *Exp Clin Cardiol.* 2013 Spring; 18(2): 129–138.

Bova, C., Sanchez, O., Prandoni, P., Lankeit, M., Konstantinides, S., Vanni, S., Jiménez, D. Identification of intermediate-risk patients with acute symptomatic pulmonary embolism. *Eur Respir J.* 2014; 44:694–703.

Chen, X., Shao, X., Zhang, Y., Zhang, Z., Tao, X., Zhai, Z., Wang, C. Assessment of the Bova score for risk stratification of acute normotensive pulmonary embolism: a systematic review and meta-analysis. *Thromb Res.* 2020; 193: 99–106.

Chopard, R., Jimenez, D., Serzian, G., Ecarnot, F., Falvo, N., Kalbacher, E., Bonnet, B., Capellier, G., Schiele, F., Bertoletti, L., Monreal, M., and Meneveau N. Renal dysfunction improves risk stratification and may call for a change in the management of intermediate- and high-risk acute pulmonary embolism: results from a multicenter cohort study with external validation. *Crit Care.* 2021; 25:1–11.

Dellas, C., Puls, M., Lankeit, M., Schäfer, K., Cuny, M., Berner, M., Hasenfuss, G., Konstantinides, S. Elevated heart-type fatty acid-binding protein levels on admission predict an adverse outcome in normotensive patients with acute pulmonary embolism. *J Am Coll Cardiol.* 2010; 55:2150–2157.

Dunn, A. S. ACP Journal Club. The simplified Pulmonary Embolism Severity Index and high-sensitivity troponin T predicted prognosis in PE. *Ann Intern Med.* 2012; 156: JC4-12.

Ebner, M., Pagel, C. F., Sentler, C., Harjola, V. P., Bueno, H., Lerchbaumer, M. H., Stangl, K., Pieske, B., Hasenfuß, G., Konstantinides, S. V., Lankeit, M. Venous lactate improves the prediction of in-hospital adverse outcomes in normotensive pulmonary embolism. *Eur J Intern Med.* 2021; 86:25–31.

El-Menyar, A., Asim, M., Nabir, S., Ahmed, M. N., and Al-Thani, H. Implications of elevated cardiac troponin in patients presenting with acute pulmonary embolism: an observational study. *J Thorac Dis.* 2019 Aug; 11(8): 3302–3314.

Ergan, B., Ergün, R., Çalışkan, T., Aydın, K., Tokur, M. E., Savran, Y., Koca, U., Cömert, B., Gökmen, N. Mortality related risk factors in high-risk pulmonary embolism in the ICU. *Can Respir J.* 2016; 2016: 2432808.

Fernández, C., Bova, C., Sanchez, O., Prandoni, P., Lankeit, M., Konstantinides, S., Vanni, S., Fernández-Golfín, C., Yusen, R. D., Jiménez, D. Validation of a model for identification of patients at intermediate to high risk for complications associated with acute symptomatic pulmonary embolism. *Chest.* 2015; 148:211–218.

Folsom, A. R., Lutsey, P. L., Nambi, V., deFilippi, C. R., Heckbert, S. R., Cushman, M, and Ballantyne, C. M. Troponin T, NT-pro BNP, and venous thromboembolism: The Longitudinal Investigation of Thromboembolism Etiology (LITE). *Vasc Med.* 2014 Feb; 19(1): 33–41.

Frederikus, A. K., Klok and Huisman, M. V. When I treat a patient with acute pulmonary embolism at home. *Am Soc Hematol Educ Program.* 2020 Dec 4; 2020(1): 190–194.

Goldhaber, S. Z., Visani, L., De Rosa, M. Acute pulmonary embolism: clinical outcomes in the International Cooperative Pulmonary Embolism Registry (ICOPER), *Lancet.* 1999; 353:1386–1389.

Grifoni, S., Olivotto, I., Cecchini, P., Pieralli, F., Camaiti, A., Santoro, G., Conti, A., Agnelli, G., Berni, G. Short-term clinical outcome of patients with acute pulmonary embolism, normal blood pressure, and echocardiographic right ventricular dysfunction. *Circ.* 2000; 101:2817–2822.

Hellenkamp, K., Schwung, J., Rossmann, H., Kaeberich, A., Wachter, R., Hasenfuß, G., Konstantinides, S., Lankeit, M. Risk stratification of normotensive pulmonary embolism: prognostic impact of copeptin. *Eur Respir J.* 2015; 46:1701–1710.

Jiménez, D., Aujesky, D., Moores, L., Gómez, V., Lobo, J. L., Uresandi, F., Otero, R., Monreal, M., Muriel, A., Yusen, R. D. RIETE Investigators: simplification of the pulmonary embolism severity index for prognostication in patients with acute symptomatic pulmonary embolism. *Arch Intern Med.* 2010; 9;170(15):1383–1389.

Jiménez, D., Uresandi, F., Otero, R., Lobo, J. L., Monreal, M., Martí, D., Zamora, J., Muriel, A., Aujesky, D., Yusen, R. D. Troponin-based risk stratification of patients with acute nonmassive pulmonary embolism: systematic review and metanalysis. *Chest.* 2009; 136:974–982.

Konstantinides, S. V., Meyer, G., Becattini, C., Bueno, H., Geersing, G. J., Harjola, V. P., Huisman, M. V., Humbert, M., Jennings, C. S., Jiménez, D., Kucher, N., Lang, I. M., Lankeit, M., Lorusso, R., Mazzolai, L., Meneveau, N., Áinle, F. N., Prandoni, P., Pruszczyk, P., Righini, M, Torbicki, A., Belle, E. V., Zamorano, J. L.; ESC Scientific Document Group. ESC guidelines for the diagnosis and management of acute pulmonary embolism developed in collaboration with the European Respiratory Society (ERS). *Eur Heart J.* 2020 Jan 21; 41(4):543-603.

Kumamaru, K. K., George, E., Ghosh, N., Quesada, C. G., Wake, N., Gerhard-Herman, M., Rybicki, F. J. Normal ventricular diameter ratio on CT provides adequate assessment for critical right ventricular strain among patients with acute pulmonary embolism. *Int J Cardiovasc Imaging.* 2016 Jul; 32(7):1153-61.

Lankeit, M., Jiménez, D., Kostrubiec, M., Dellas, C., Kuhnert, K., Hasenfuß, G., Pruszczyk, P., Konstantinides, S., Validation of N-terminal pro-brain natriuretic peptide cut-off values for risk stratification of pulmonary embolism. *Eur Respir J.* 2014; 43: 1669-1677.

Laporte, S., Mismetti, P., Décousus, H., Uresandi, F., Otero, R., Lobo, J. L., Monreal, M., The RIETE investigators vlinical predictors for fatal pulmonary embolism in 15,520 patients with venous thromboembolism: findings from the Registro Informatizado de la Enfermedad TromboEmbolica venosa (RIETE) Registry. *Circ.* 2008; 117:1711–1716.

Lega, J. C., Lacasse, Y., Lakhal L., Provencher, S. Natriuretic peptides and troponins in pulmonary embolism: a meta-analysis. *Thorax.* 2009 Oct; 64 (10):869-75.

Leidi, A., Bex, S., Righini, M., Berner, A., Grosgurin, O., Marti, C. Risk stratification in patients with acute pulmonary embolism: current evidence and perspectives. J Clin Med. 2022 May; 11(9): 2533.

Mirambeaux, R., León, F., Bikdeli, B., Morillo, R., Barrios, D., Mercedes, E., Moores, L., Tapson, V., Yusen, R. D., Jiménez, D. Intermediate-high risk pulmonary embolism. *TH Open.* 2019 Oct; 3(4): e356–e363.

Morrone, D., Morrone, V., Acute Pulmonary Embolism: focus on the clinical picture. *Korean Circ J.* 2018 May; 48(5): 365–381.

Nithianandan, H., Reilly, A., Tritschler, T., Wells, P. Applying rigorous eligibility criteria to studies evaluating prognostic utility of serum biomarkers in pulmonary embolism: a systematic review and meta-analysis. *Thromb Res.* 2020; 195:195–208.

Ocak, G, Vossen, C. Y., Verduijn, M., Dekker, F. W., Rosendaal, F. R., Cannegieter, S. C., Lijfering, W. M. Risk of venous thrombosis in patients with major illnesses: results from the MEGA study. *J Thromb Haemost.* 2013; 11:116–23.

Pollack, C. V., Schreiber, D., Goldhaber, S, Z., Slattery, D., Fanikos, J., O'Neil B. J., Thompson, J. R., Hiestand, B., Briese, B. A., Pendleton, R. C., Miller, C. D., Kline, J. A. Clinical characteristics, management, and outcomes of patients diagnosed with acute pulmonary embolism in the emergency department initial report of EMPEROR (Multicenter Emergency Medicine Pulmonary Embolism in the Real World Registry) *J Am Coll Cardiol.* 2011; 57(6):700–706.

Quezada, A., Jiménez, D., Bikdeli, B., Moores, L., Porres-Aguilar, M., Aramberri, M., Lima, J., Ballaz, A., Yusen, R. D., Monreal, M. Systolic blood pressure and mortality in acute symptomatic pulmonary embolism. *Int J Cardiol.* 2019; 302:157–163.

Silvy, L., Patrick, M., Herve, D. Uresandi, F., Otero, R., Lobo, J. L, Monreal, M. Clinical predictors for fatal pulmonary embolism in 15,520 patients with venous thromboembolism - findings from the Registro Informatizado de la Enfermedad TromboEmbolica venosa (RIETE) registry. *Circ.* 2008; 117(13):1711–1716

Torbicki, A., Galie, N., Covezzoli, A., Rossi E., De Rossa, M, Goldhaber, S. Z. Right heart thrombi in pulmonary embolism - results from the International Cooperative Pulmonary Embolism Registry. *J Am Coll Cardiol.* 2003; 41(12):2245–2251.

Vanni, S., Socci, F., Pepe, G., Nazerian, P., Viviani, G., Baioni, M., Conti, A., Grifoni, S. High plasma lactate levels are associated with increased risk of in-hospital mortality in patients with pulmonary embolism. *Acad Emerg Med.* 2011; 18:830–835.

Vanni, S., Viviani, G., Baioni, M., Pepe, G., Nazerian, P., Socci. F., Bartolucci M., Bartolini, M., Grifoni, M. Prognostic value of plasma lactate levels among patients with acute pulmonary embolism: the thrombo-embolism lactate outcome study. *Ann Emerg Med.* 2013 Mar; 61(3):330-8.

Zhai Z., Wang, D., Lei, J., Yang, Y., Xu, X., Ji, Y., Yi, Q., Chen, H., Hu, X., Liu, Z., Zhai. Z., Wang, D. Lei, J., Yang, Y., Xiaomao X., Yingqun, J. Yi, Q., Chen, H., Hu, X., Liu Z., Mao Y., Zhang J., Shi, J., Zhang, Z., Wu, S., Gao, Q., Tao, X., Xie, W., Wan, J. Zhang, Y., Zhang S., Zhen, K., Zhonghe Zhang, Z., Fang, B. Wang, C. Trends in risk stratification, in-hospital management and mortality of patients with acute pulmonary embolism: An analysis from the China pulmonary thromboembolism Registry Study (CURES) *Eur Respir J.* 2021; 58:2002963.

Zhou, X. Y., Ben, S. Q., Chen, H. L., and Ni, S. S. The prognostic value of pulmonary embolism severity index in acute pulmonary embolism: a meta-analysis. *Respir Res.* 2012; 13(1): 111.

Zondag, W., Mos, I. C., Creemers-Schild, D., Hoogerbrugge, A. D. M., Dekkers, O. M., Dolsma, J., Eijsvogel M., Faber, L. M, Hofstee, H. N. A, Hovens, M. M. C., Jonkers, G. J. P. M., Van Kralingen, K. W., Kruip, M. J. H. A, T Vlasveld T., De Vreede, M. J. M, Huisman, M. V.; Outpatient treatment in patients with acute pulmonary embolism: the Hestia Study. *J Thromb Haemost.* 2011;9(8):1500–1507.

Chapter 4

Non-Invasive Imaging in Acute Pulmonary Embolism

Elizabeta Srbinovska Kostovska*, **PhD**
University Cardiology Clinic, Clinical Center, Medical Faculty,
University "St Cyril and Metodij" Skopje, North Macedonia

Abstract

Pulmonary embolism (PE) is a condition that can lead to acute heart failure (AHF). In critical and emergency settings, echocardiography is crucial in providing patients with important, often lifesaving information. Identifying high-risk patients with suspected or confirmed PE and assessing their risk of early mortality is of utmost importance. Emergency computed tomography pulmonary angiography (CTPA) or bedside echocardiography, depending on availability and clinical condition, are recommended for suspected high-risk patients with PE and hemodynamic instability. Echocardiography can detect right ventricular (RV) pressure overload and dysfunction caused by PE. Several echocardiographic parameters, as per the diagnosis and treatment guidelines for PE, can indicate its presence and severity. These parameters include right ventricular enlargement, RV basal diameter greater than the left ventricle (LV) with a ratio larger than 1 on a four-chamber view, McConnell's sign, and sign 60/60. PE-induced RV overload leads to impaired LV function, resulting in septal flattening and D-shape of the LV. Estimating the severity of pulmonary hypertension in PE patients involves assessing the velocity of tricuspid regurgitation and the size and collapsibility of the vena cava. However, in some cases, the velocity alone may not be sufficient for estimating pulmonary

* Corresponding Author's Email: esrbinovska@yahoo.com.

In: Pulmonary Embolism
Editors: Irena Mitevska, Sonja Salinger, Marijan Bosevski et al.
ISBN: 979-8-89113-175-0

hypertension, necessitating further information about tricuspid regurgitation shape, density, and timing in relation to its severity. Predisposing factors, such as mobile thrombus in the truncus of the pulmonary artery and right heart chambers, can aid in diagnosing PE. However, echocardiography does not play a central role in suspected PE patients without hemodynamic instability (obstruction of smaller branches of the pulmonary artery with smaller RV overload). In such cases, clinical judgment, predictive scores, predisposing factors, and blood tests (D-dimer) are crucial, with CTPA being a more sensitive method for diagnosing PE. It is important to note that negative echocardiography results cannot exclude PE, as signs of RV overload and dysfunction can also be present due to concomitant cardiac or respiratory diseases.

Keywords: acute pulmonary embolism, pulmonary hypertension, computed tomography, echocardiography, right ventricular enlargement

Introduction

Multimodality cardiovascular imaging, primarily echocardiography (TTE) and computed tomography pulmonary angiography (CTPA) are essential approaches for the prompt and accurate diagnosis of acute pulmonary embolism (PE). They play a vital role in evaluating the hemodynamic significance of PE, guiding clinical decision-making, determining therapeutic strategies, and assessing therapeutic efficacy in the post-acute phase of PE. Having a high clinical suspicion, recognizing abrupt onset symptoms, and identifying predisposing factors for PE are key factors in establishing a timely diagnosis. Additionally, selecting the most appropriate cardiovascular imaging modality is crucial for an effective diagnostic process.

Acute pulmonary embolism is one of the conditions that can lead to acute heart failure (AHF). Alongside PE, other conditions that can cause AHF include acute coronary syndrome, hypertension emergency, arrhythmias, mechanical causes of acute heart failure, infection, and tamponade (Figure 1). In critical and emergency settings, echocardiography is crucial in providing patients essential, often lifesaving, information. According to the Guidelines for the Diagnosis and Management of Acute Pulmonary Embolism, conducting an initial risk stratification of suspected and confirmed PE in patients with hemodynamic instability is highly important. This allows for identifying patients at high risk of early mortality (Konstantinides et al., 2020; McDonagh et al., 2021).

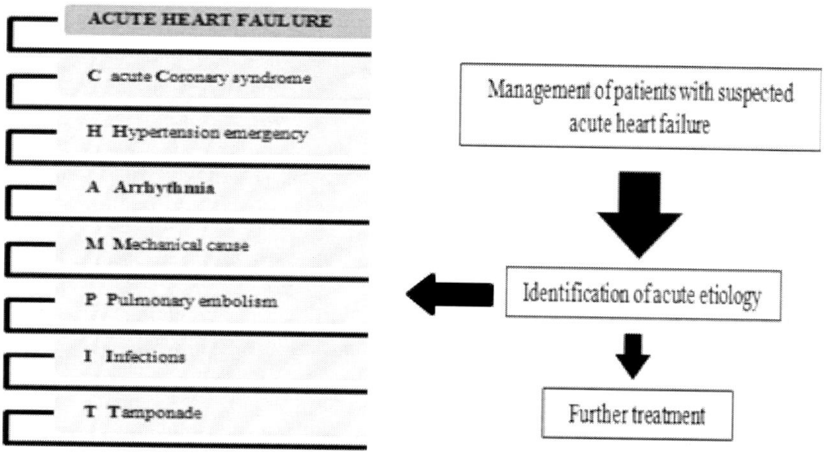

Figure 1. Initial strategy in acute heart failure (Adapted from McDonagh, 2021).

High-risk PE patients necessitate an immediate diagnostic and therapeutic approach due to their critical condition. Cardiac instability in these cases may manifest as cardiac arrest requiring cardiopulmonary resuscitation, obstructive shock, or persistent hypotension. For suspected high-risk patients with PE and hemodynamic instability, it is recommended to perform bedside echocardiography or emergency CT, depending on the availability at the medical facility and the patient's clinical condition. Bedside echocardiography is feasible in any setting and is particularly well-suited for use with acutely ill or severely compromised patients.

The pathophysiological events during acute pulmonary thromboembolism, resulting from anatomical obstruction of the affected pulmonary area and induced vasoconstriction, leading to an acute increase in pulmonary vascular resistance (PVR) and the development of increased pulmonary arterial pressure (PAP). These changes contribute to right ventricular (RV) afterload, leading to RV dilatation and dysfunction. The elevated RV afterload causes increased RV wall stress, leading to RV ischemia, reduced RV contractility, and further reductions in RV output. Consequently, RV dilatation causes the interventricular septum to bow into the LV, impairing LV filling and decreasing LV contractility and cardiac output. Additionally, increased RV afterload results in the dilatation of the tricuspid annulus with varying degrees of disturbed coaptation of the tricuspid valve, leading to significant tricuspid regurgitation. The severity of tricuspid regurgitation can be used to calculate pulmonary hypertension (Hockstein et al., 2021; Quintero-Martinez et al., 2022). Echocardiography can detect these hemodynamic changes to varying degrees depending on their expression (Bryce et al., 2019; Cohen et al., 2012; Konstantinidis et al., 2020).

If bedside echocardiography reveals RV dilatation and dysfunction even without CT, prompt treatment for high-risk PE patients can be initiated in patients with hemodynamic instability. However, in cases where there is no RV dilatation and dysfunction, alternative causes of shock or hemodynamic instability must be investigated. CTPA is generally an accurate diagnostic tool for acute pulmonary embolism and is considered the gold standard for evaluating patients with suspected PE (Figure 2). Nevertheless, there are situations where the clinical condition of patients precludes the performance of CTPA, or the procedure may not be available at the institution, presenting challenges for conducting it.

Table 1. Recommendation for diagnosis of pulmonary embolism (adapted from Konstantinides et al., 2020)

Recommendations	Class	Level
Suspected PE with hemodynamic instability		
In suspected high-risk PE, as indicated by the presence of hemodynamic instability, bedside echocardiography or emergency CTPA (depending on availability and clinical circumstances) is recommended for diagnosis.	I	C
CTPA		
It is recommended to reject the diagnosis of PE (without further testing) if CTPA is normal in a patient with low or intermediate clinical probability or who is PE-unlikely.	I	A
It is recommended to accept the diagnosis of PE (without further testing) if CTPA shows segmental or more proximal filling defects in a patient with intermediate or high clinical probability.	I	B
It should be considered to reject the diagnosis of PE (without further testing) if CTPA is normal in a patient with high clinical probability or who is PE-likely.	IIa	B
Ventilation perfusion scintigraphy		
It is recommended to reject the diagnosis of PE (without further testing) if the perfusion lung scan is normal.	I	A

Current guidelines recommend performing CTPA in patients with a high suspicion of PE and hemodynamic instability. If CTPA reveals segmental or more proximal filling defects in patients with intermediate or high-risk clinical probability, the diagnosis of PE is accepted without further testing. Conversely, if CTPA is normal in patients with low or intermediate clinical probability or those deemed unlikely to have PE, the diagnosis of PE is rejected. The same applies to patients with a high clinical probability or those considered PE-likely (Table 1) (Bossone et al., 2013; Dahhan et al., 2016; Hockstein et al., 2021; Konstantinidis et al., 2020; Poor et al., 2023).

However, the absence of hemodynamic instability does not rule out the diagnosis of PE or the possibility of the occurrence and progression of RV dysfunction. The echocardiographic findings in patients depend on the level of obstruction in the pulmonary artery and bronchi. In cases of obstruction in the smaller pulmonary artery branches, where RV overload is less pronounced, echocardiography plays a less central role. Therefore, it becomes crucial to stratify patients suspected of having PE without hemodynamic instability into intermediate and low-risk categories for PE. In such situations, a comprehensive assessment of clinical probability using all predictive scores is necessary, along with estimating additional parameters like risk factors or predisposing factors for PE, biomarkers (such as D-dimer), and co-morbidities (Figure 3).

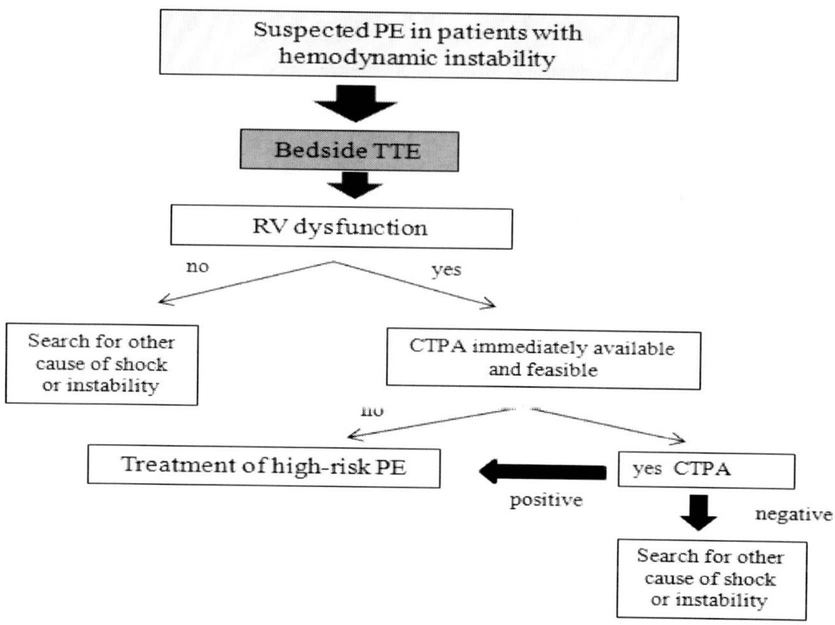

Figure 2. Algorithm for PE diagnosis in patients suspected of PE with hemodynamic instability (adapted from Konstantinides et al., 2020).

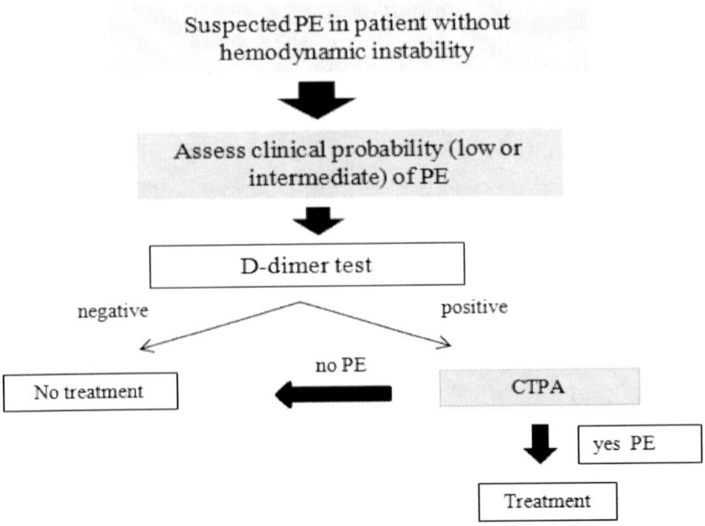

Figure 3. Algorithm for PE diagnosis in patients suspected of PE without hemodynamic instability (adapted from Konstantinides et al., 2020).

It is essential to remember that echocardiography has a negative predictive value of 40–50%, meaning that negative results cannot definitively exclude the presence of PE. Another imaging modality that can aid in identifying patients with acute PE is the ventilation/perfusion (V/Q) scan. If the perfusion scan yields negative results, the diagnosis of acute PE can be ruled out (Table 1) (Konstantinides et al., 2020).

Role of Cardiovascular Imaging Modalities in the Diagnosis of Pulmonary Embolism

CTPA and transthoracic echocardiography are crucial imaging modalities for diagnosing PE and evaluating its hemodynamic significance. The information obtained from these imaging studies plays a vital role in determining the appropriate therapeutic strategy and assessing the therapeutic efficiency and prognosis of patients with PE. Each imaging modality has its own set of advantages and disadvantages when diagnosing patients with acute PE and assessing disease severity, as shown in Table 2.

Table 2. Advantages and disadvantages of the cardiovascular imaging modalities in assessing pulmonary embolism (adapted from Kim et al., 2021)

Imaging modalities	Advantage	Disadvantage
TTE	Possibility of bedside evaluation	Cannot identify the thrombus extent
	assessment of hemodynamics	High sensitivity, low specificity
	relatively low costs	Suboptimal in patients with poor imaging window
	widely available	
	no radiation	
CTPA	High positive predictive value	radiation
	High diagnostic accuracy	contraindication in advanced renal disease (contrast agent)
	Imaging modality of choice	
	Direct visualization of the thrombus	
	Possible assessment of other cardiac structures	
	Superior spatial resolution and multiplanar reconstruction	
Ventilation perfusion scan	High diagnostic accuracy	limited availability
	Can distinguish CTEPH from PE	radiation
MRI	free from ionizing radiation information for cardiac structure and flow mechanics	limited availability contraindication in advanced renal disease (gadolinium)

TTE – transthoracic echocardiography; CTPA – computed tomography pulmonary angiography; MRI – magnetic resonance; CTEPH – chronic thromboembolic pulmonary hypertension.

Computed Tomography Pulmonary Angiography

CTPA is the method of choice for diagnosing patients with PE, demonstrating a sensitivity of 83% and specificity of 96%. The available data suggest that a negative CTPA result is a reliable criterion for excluding PE in patients with a low or intermediate clinical probability of PE. However, further investigation is warranted in cases where patients have a negative CTPA result but a high clinical probability. The Prospective Investigation of Pulmonary Embolism II trial (PIOPED II) yielded noteworthy results, showing that CTPA has a high negative predictive value (96%) for patients with a low clinical probability of PE and a high positive predictive value (96%) for patients with a high clinical probability of PE (Stein et al., 2006).

CTPA enables the assessment of the presence, location, and degree of thrombi, as well as the total number of involved pulmonary vascular segments and the degree of embolic obstruction. CTPE allows determining the total number of pulmonary vascular segments obstructed by embolic events. Various scoring systems exist to assess the severity of the current episode of PE by quantifying pulmonary angiography (PA) clot loads. One such scoring system is the Qanadli score, which considers the number of obstructed arterial segments and the degree of vascular obstruction. In some studies, this score has been reported as a reliable predictor of RV dysfunction or mortality (Qanadli et al., 2001; Vedovati et al., 2013).

Acute emboli are commonly found at vessel bifurcations and may lead to complete or partial artery obstruction. Complete obstruction manifests as a hypoattenuating contrast defect that involves the entire lumen while often maintaining a normal vessel diameter. Distal infarcts caused by complete obstruction appear as triangular subpleural consolidations or ground-glass opacities (Figure 4). On the other hand, partial obstructions can be central or eccentric. In patients with chronic obstructive PE, PTCA changes differ from those observed in acute PE, with identifiable obstructions and a narrowed vessel diameter distal to the obstruction. CTPA is critical in differentiating acute from chronic thromboembolic disease (Kim et al., 2021; Poor et al., 2023).

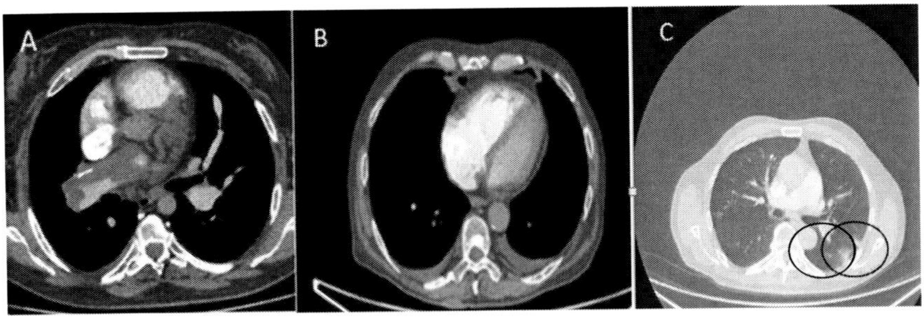

Figure 4. Computed tomography pulmonary angiography showing (A) large filling defects resulting in near total occlusion of the right pulmonary artery and (B) right heart dilatation which is greater than left ventricular dimension with small pleural effusion bilaterally; (C) Sub pleural ischemic wedge-shaped consolidative changes on the posterior basal left side.

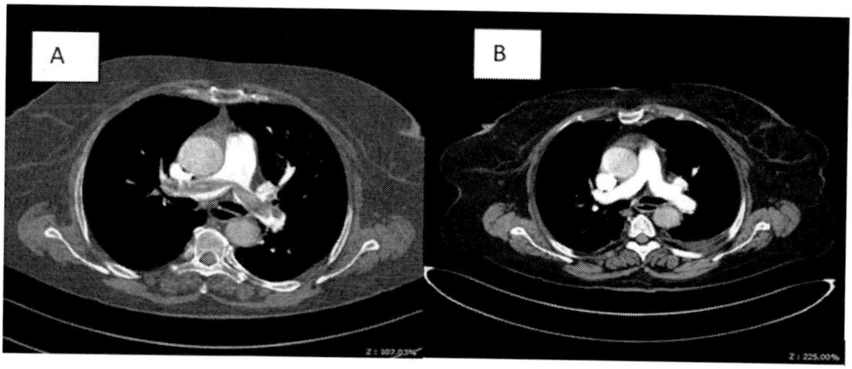

Figure 5. A big"saddle" thrombus at the bifurcation of the pulmonary artery on CTPA (A) and the CTPA after PE treatment (B).

CTPA can provide valuable information about the hemodynamic significance of PE, such as right heart dilatation, which suggests RV dysfunction. One commonly used marker for RV dysfunction is the RV/LV ratio, which can be measured from CTPA images. In published meta-analyses, a ratio greater than 0.9–1 has been identified as a reliable indicator of RV dysfunction. This parameter, RV/LV ratio, predicts mortality in patients with PE based on CTPA measurements. Additionally, leftward ventricular septal bowing and contrast reflux into the inferior vena cava are other parameters that may suggest RV dysfunction in patients with PE. However, these parameters have shown lower sensitivity and specificity compared to the RV/LV ratio (Becattini et al., 2011; Seon et al., 2011; Schoepf et al., 2004).

CTPA offers numerous advantages, including high accuracy and predictive value and the possibility of superior spatial resolution and multiplanar reconstruction. Wide array CT technology provides a substantial length per rotation, effectively reducing motion artifacts. Dual-energy CT has proven beneficial in enhancing the sensitivity of perfusion defects, enabling salvaging of suboptimal studies, and reducing contrast exposure to patients (Farag et al., 2022; Konstantinides et al., 2020; Morris et al., 2022; Stein et al., 2006).

CTPA can also be utilized to evaluate therapeutic results, representing another important role of this imaging modality in assessing these patients (Figure 5).

Transthoracic Echocardiography

Echocardiography serves as a quick and straightforward method for risk stratification of patients suspected of PE and is crucial in guiding treatment strategies. By examining the pathophysiological cascade of acute PE, transthoracic echocardiography (TEE) can help reveal the progressive deterioration of the clinical condition and the hemodynamic significance of acute PE. TEE allows for the monitoring of patients with pulmonary thromboembolism, enabling the detection of RV dilatation, assessment of tricuspid regurgitation and the development of pulmonary hypertension, identification of deep veins (DV) overload and decrease in RV contractility, and estimation of RV function, as well as changes in LV function (Dabbouseh et al., 2019; Kim et al., 2021; Konstantinides et al., 2020; Kucher et al., 2005; Lee et al., 2008; Park et al., 2023; Rudinski et al., 2010).

According to the Guideline of Diagnosis and Treatment of PE, several echocardiographic parameters may be observed, and their presence and expression can vary in patients with PE. These parameters include right ventricular enlargement, with the basal diameter of the RV larger than the LV and a ratio greater than 1 on the four-chamber view. Other indicators, such as MC Connell's and 60/60 signs, can also be seen in patients with PE. RV overload, which occurs during PE, leads to impaired left ventricular function, resulting in septal flattening and a D-shaped appearance of the LV. The velocity of tricuspid regurgitation and the size and collapsibility of the vena cava are parameters used to estimate the severity of present pulmonary hypertension in patients with PE (Bossone et al., 2013; Konstantinides et al., 2020; Lopez-Candales et al., 2008; Zaidi et al., 2021).

The presence of RV dysfunction in patients with PE correlates with high-risk patients and is an independent predictor of a poor outcome. RV enlargement is considered present when the basal diameter of the RV exceeds that of the LV, resulting in an RV/LV ratio greater than 1 on the four-chamber view, along with an index of the eccentricity of the left ventricle (LV) in the short axis greater than RV, which occurs during PE. The RV overload leads to impaired left ventricular function, resulting in septal flattening and a D-shaped appearance of the LV (Figure 6).

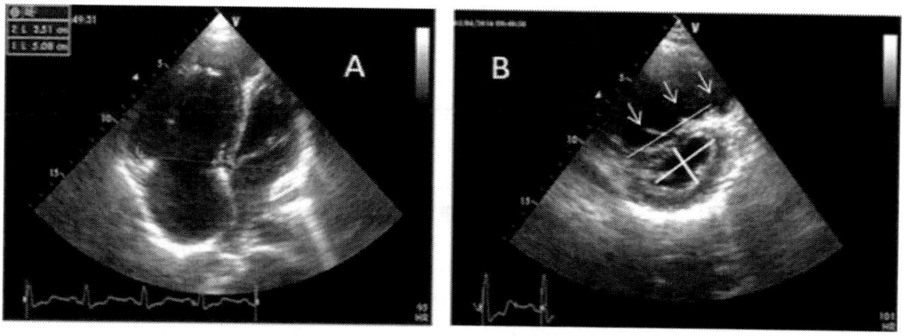

Figure 6. Transthoracic echocardiography of (A) four-chamber view showing that the right ventricle is bigger than the left ventricle, and the ratio RV/LV is bigger than 1; (B) Parasternal short axis at the level of the papillary muscles showing dilated right ventricle with flattening of the interventricular septum (D-shape of the left ventricle) and index of the eccentricity of the left ventricle bigger than 1.

McConnell's sign, characterized by hypokinesis of the RV free wall and hyperdynamic apex, can be observed in patients with PE, with a sensitivity of 77% and a specificity of 95%. One of the presumed mechanisms for this sign is the normal LV pulling on the apex of the heart. However, it is essential to note that this sign is not pathognomonic for PE, as it can also be seen in patients with RV infarction in a similar percentage. RV hypokinesis is considered a poor prognostic indicator for survival in patients with PE (McConnell et al., 1996) (Figure 7).

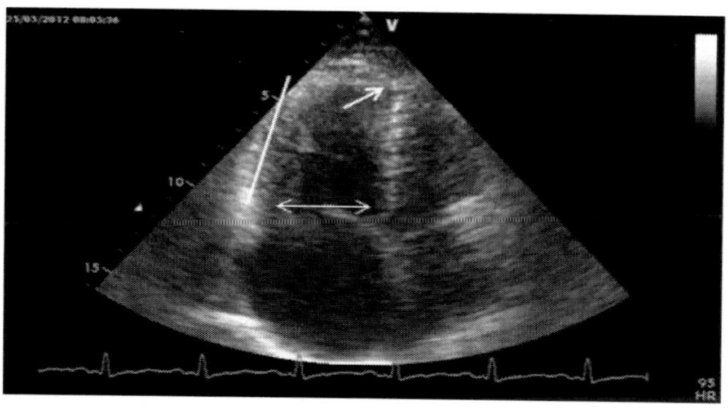

Figure 7. Transthoracic four-chamber echocardiography with a typical configuration is very often observed in patients with acute PE due to the decrease in the contractility of the free wall of the right ventricle and the hyperdynamic apex (McConnell's sign). The described changes are visible in real-time.

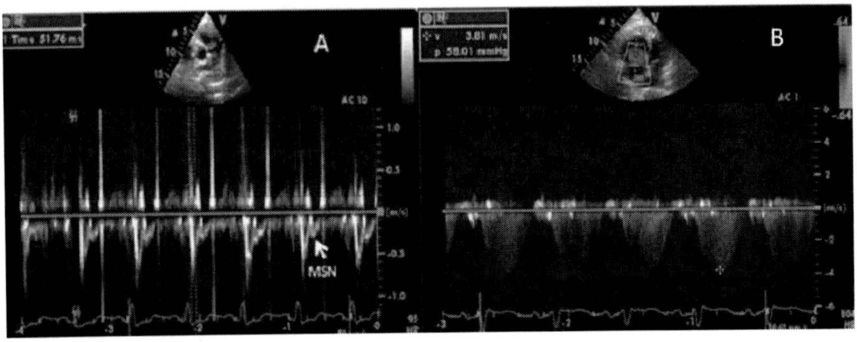

Figure 8. (A) Pulsed Doppler echocardiography in RV outflow truck showing acceleration time of the pulmonary artery less than 60msec and there is the presence of mid-systolic notch (MSN). (B) Continuous Doppler showing peak systolic velocity of the tricuspid regurgitation bigger than 3.8 m/s.

Another important parameter is the "60/60 sign." The first "60" refers to the acceleration time derived from pulsed Doppler in the RV outflow tract, which is less than 60 msec and is accompanied by the presence of a mid-systolic notch. The second "60" pertains to the peak systolic gradient obtained from tricuspid regurgitation, with a peak velocity greater than 3.8 m/s (Figure 8).

The velocity of tricuspid regurgitation (TR) and the size and collapsibility of the vena cava by more than 50% are parameters used to estimate the severity of pulmonary hypertension in patients with PE. However, relying solely on TR velocity may not always be sufficient to assess pulmonary hypertension accurately. Additional information about the shape, density, and timing of TR during systole is necessary to avoid underestimation (e.g., in patients with severe TR) or overestimation (e.g., in patients with high cardiac output) of pulmonary hypertension.

Furthermore, misinterpretation of TR can occur in cases of artifacts from tricuspid valve closure or poor image quality, leading to confusion with the tricuspid regurgitant jet. To monitor these patients and assess the improvement of their clinical and objective condition after PE, a reduction in estimated pulmonary hypertension can serve as a useful parameter (An et al., 2022; Humbert et al., 2022).

Estimation of the systolic pulmonary artery pressure (sPAP) is based on a formula that incorporates the peak velocity of TR (vTR) and the right atrial pressure (RAP). The RAP is estimated using the dimensions and collapsibility of the vena cava (Table 3). The formula for estimating sPAP is as follows: $sPAP = 4 \times (vTR)^2 + \text{estimated RAP}$.

Table 3. Estimation of right atrial pressure (Humbert M et al., 2022)

Dimension of v. cava inferior	Collapsibility of v. cava inferior	Right atrial pressure (mmHg)
<2.1 cm	>50%	3 (0–5)
>2.1 cm	>50%	8 (5–10)
>2.1 cm	<50%	15 (10–12)

Estimating and monitoring RV function in patients with PE during the acute phase and after recovery is crucial. Echocardiography provides recommended parameters for assessing RV function, such as tricuspid annular plane systolic excursion (TAPSE) using M-mode, peak systolic velocity of the tricuspid annulus via Tissue Doppler imaging, and estimation of the global longitudinal strain on the RV using speckle tracking (GLS). These parameters offer valuable insights into the longitudinal function of the RV. If TAPSE is less than 17 mm, S wave is less than 9.5 cm/s, and GLS is less than -20%, according to vendor cut-off values, it highly suggests RV dysfunction.

By employing 2D speckle tracking, we can estimate both global and regional RV functions. A GLS lower than 19 is an unfavorable prognostic indicator for the prognosis and survival of PE patients. Additionally, we can assess global RV systolic function by estimating functional area change (FAC). An RV FAC of <35% indicates RV systolic dysfunction. Three-dimensional echocardiography (3D) allows for estimating RV ejection fraction (EF), a globally validated measure of RV systolic function, providing more precise parameters and being the recommended method for estimating RV EF compared to CMR.

Derived parameters such as the right myocardial performance index (RIMP) or Tei index can be determined by pulse Doppler or Tissue Doppler imaging (TDI) and serve as indices of global RV function. An >0.43 by pulsed-wave Doppler and >0.54 by TDI indicate RV dysfunction. A meta-analysis of 30-day mortality demonstrated that RV dysfunction is a significant prognostic parameter in PE patients. As independent predictors, Echocardiographic parameters are easily investigated and emphasize various measurements, combinations of echocardiographic parameters, and risk scores as prognostic factors.

Echocardiography enables the straightforward assessment of disease severity and patient follow-up while providing crucial prognostic information about RV function and pulmonary hypertension (Alerhand et al., 2021; Barco et al., 2019; Bosevski et al., 2018; Cho et al., 2014; Jones et al., 2019; Lung et al., 2015; Srbinovska Kostovska E., 2013; Vamsidhar et al., 2017).

Predisposing factors, including mobile thrombus in the right atrium (RA) and right ventricle (RV), thrombus in the vena cava, and the pulmonary artery truncus, can aid in the diagnostic process. However, TTE often faces limitations in visualizing the precise location or extent of pulmonary thrombi or emboli. Three-dimensional echocardiography (3D) offers enhanced possibilities to identify thrombi, particularly in the main truncus of the pulmonary artery (Figure 9). A thrombus in the right heart is also associated with a poorer survival rate.

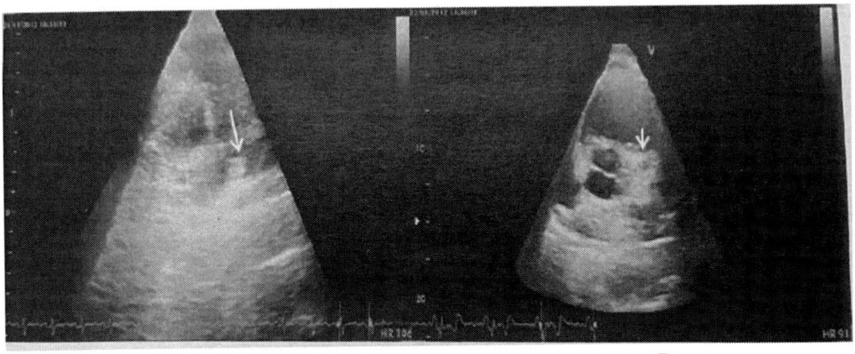

A B

Figure 9. Three-dimensional echocardiography. (A) Thrombus at the bifurcation of the pulmonary artery; (B) Thrombus just below the pulmonary valve (Courtesy of Elizabeta Srbinovska Kostovska).

Signs of RV overload and dysfunction may also be present in the absence of acute PE and could be attributed to concomitant cardiac or respiratory conditions. As a result, achieving an accurate and timely diagnosis of acute PE requires consideration of the patient's clinical presentation, predisposing factors, predictive scores, and a careful evaluation of the advantages and limitations of various imaging modalities.

Transesophageal Echocardiography

Transesophageal echocardiography (TEE) is crucial in critically ill patients with suboptimal TTE image quality. TEE enables the exclusion of other potential diagnoses at the bedside, particularly in severely unstable patients with respiratory and hemodynamic distress. In cases with a high clinical probability of PE and dilatation of the RV, initiating specific therapeutic agents based on TEE findings can lead to excellent clinical outcomes. CTPA can be performed later, once the patient's critical condition has stabilized, to further support the decision for specific therapy initiation (Bacallado et al., 2019).

Ventilation/Perfusion Scintigraphy

Ventilation/perfusion scanning is an established diagnostic test for suspected PE patients, but it is currently reserved for individuals who cannot undergo a CT scan (e.g., due to size constraints), those with renal failure, pregnant patients, or individuals with contrast allergies. In cases of acute PE, perfusion defects are observed without corresponding ventilation defects. According to current guidelines, PE can be excluded when the study is classified as normal and confirmed when the study is classified as high probability. However, it is essential to consider that other conditions can also lead to V/Q mismatches, such as veno-occlusive disorders, vasculitis, congenital pulmonary vascular abnormalities, pulmonary artery sarcoma, fibrosing mediastinitis, malignancy, and mediastinal lymphadenopathy (Konstantinides et al., 2014; Kim et al., 2021).

V/Q scanning remains an important diagnostic tool, especially in conjunction with CTPA, for discriminating between chronic thromboembolic pulmonary hypertension (CTEPH) and acute PE patients (Humbert et al., 2023; Kim et al., 2021).

Magnetic Resonance Pulmonary Angiography

Magnetic resonance pulmonary angiography (MRPA) can offer valuable insights into the morphological and functional changes in patients with PE, including vascular filling defects, complete absence of vessel enhancement, and pulmonary artery dilatation. However, MRPA exhibits lower sensitivity for detecting PE than CTPA, particularly in assessing peripheral regions. As a result, MRPA is not recommended for routine investigation of PE, and further studies are required to determine its clinical utility (Kim et al., 2021; Pleszewski et al., 2006).

Pulmonary Angiography

Pulmonary angiography (PA) offers direct visualization of obstructive vasculature or thrombi, providing superior visualization of peripheral pulmonary vessels that might go undetected with other non-invasive imaging modalities (such as CTPA or MRA). Additionally, PA allows for hemodynamic measurements. Filling defects or the loss of pulmonary arterial branches indicate PE. PA is particularly useful in patients suspected of having CTEPH. In cases where patients with acute PE present with shock or hypotension, prompt catheter-directed thrombolysis or thrombectomy can be performed following the diagnosis of acute PE (Kim et al., 2021; Konstantinides et al., 2014).

Lung Ultrasound

Lung ultrasound (LUS) is a safe and valuable bedside diagnostic tool with a significant role in the diagnostic process of critically ill patients, including those with acute PE. Some studies have demonstrated that LUS can detect subpleural pulmonary infarcts as triangular, polygonal, or rounded pleural-based, echo-poor consolidations with sharp margins, sometimes accompanied by localized pleural effusion. While LUS can aid in diagnosing PE, its sensitivity is suboptimal compared to CTPA. It is limited to cases where CTPA is contraindicated or not feasible, as subpleural infarcts may not always be present in patients with PE (Nazerian P. et al., 2022).

A negative LUS study cannot definitively rule out PE, but positive findings may help reduce the overuse of CTPA and unnecessary contrast exposure (Abdelkader et al., 2021; Nazerian et al., 2022; Squizzato et al., 2015).

Imaging Modalities in Special Cases

Imaging Diagnosis in Pregnancy

Modern imaging techniques offer low radiation exposure for maternal and fetal health. Ventilation/perfusion scans and CTPA provide fetal radiation doses well below the threshold associated with fetal radiation complications without compromising image quality. In pregnant patients, a chest X-ray may be indicated. If the X-ray is normal or inconclusive, CTPA or perfusion lung scan should be performed to exclude or confirm the presence of PE.

In cases where CTPA or lung scan yields indeterminate or positive results, low molecular weight heparin (LMWH) should be administered at a therapeutic dose. It is essential to assess the severity of PE and the risk of early death, followed by referral to a multidisciplinary team experienced in managing PE during pregnancy.

A low-dose perfusion scan can be performed for diagnosing PE, which results in lower maternal radiation exposure and offers higher diagnostic accuracy compared to CTPA (Armstrong et al., 2017; Chan et al., 2014; Wan et al., 2017).

Impaired Renal Function and Diagnosis of Pulmonary Embolism

CTPA can potentially induce radio-contrast-induced nephropathy, particularly in patients at high risk of developing renal failure, such as those with diabetes. Using gadolinium in magnetic resonance imaging can also lead to nephrogenic systemic fibrosis. In cases where patients have impaired renal function and suspected PE, a ventilation/perfusion scan is preferred over CTPA (Kim et al., 2021; Pleszewski et al., 2006).

Conclusion

Diagnosing acute PE can be challenging, and accurate identification of high clinical probability and the appropriate cardiovascular imaging modality are crucial for a prompt diagnosis, which can be lifesaving in some cases. In suspected high-risk patients with PE presenting with hemodynamic instability, emergency CTPA or bedside echocardiography is recommended, depending on availability in the institution and the patient's clinical condition.

Combining multimodality cardiovascular imaging can offer a more comprehensive perspective on the diagnosis for patients with low or intermediate risk or those with an unlikely PE. This information is essential for determining the appropriate therapeutic strategy and assessing therapeutic efficacy and prognosis in PE patients.

Each imaging modality has advantages and disadvantages in diagnosing patients with acute PE, stratifying risk, assessing disease severity, and selecting the appropriate therapeutic strategy. Additionally, these modalities play a crucial role in the follow-up of patients after an acute event. Despite technological advances and an improved understanding of predisposing factors and clinical manifestations, uncertainty still exists in diagnosing certain patients with PE.

References

Abdelkader, A. A. M., Zidan, M., Eshmawey, H., Gharraf, H.: Study for evaluation of using transthoracic lung ultrasound in diagnosis of pulmonary embolism; *European Respiratory Journal* 2021 58: PA3546.

Alerhand, S., Sundaram, T., Gottlieb, M. What are the echocardiographic findings of acute right ventricular strain that suggest pulmonary embolism? *Anaesth Crit Care Pain Med.* 2021 Apr;40(2):100852.

An, J., Nam, Y., Cho, H, Chang, J., Kim K. D., and Lee, KS. Acute Pulmonary Embolism and Chronic Tromboembolic Pulmonary Hypertension: Clinical and Serial CT Pulmonary Angiographic Features. *J. Korean Med. Sci.*, (2022) 37(10): e76.

Armstrong, L., Gleeson, F., Mackillop, L., Mutch, S., Beale, A. Survey of UK imaging practice for the investigation of pulmonary embolism in pregnancy. *Clin Radiol* 2017; 72:696701).

Bacallado, M., Izquierdo-Gómez, M. M., García-Niebla, J., Jiménez, J. J., Iribarren, J. L., Cerdeña. I. L., Lacalzada-Almeida, J. Role of echocardiography in a patient with suspected acute pulmonary embolism: a case report. *Journal of Medical Case Reports* (2019) 13:37

Barco, S., Mahmoudpour, S. H., Planquette, B., Sanchez, O., Konstantinides. S. V., Meyer, G. Prognostic value of right ventricular dysfunction or elevated cardiac biomarkers in patients with low risk pulmonary embolism: a systematic review and Meta-analysis; *European Heart Journal* (2019) 40, 902-910.

Becattini, C., Agnelli. G., Vedovati, M. C., Pruszczyk, P., Casazza, F., Grifoni, S., Salvi, A., Bianchi, M., Douma, R., Konstantinides, S., Lankeit, M., Duranti, M. Multidetector computed tomography for acute pulmonary embolism: diagnosis and risk stratification in a single test. *Eur. Heart J.* 2011; 32(13):1657-1663.

Bosevski, M., Krstevski, G., Gjorgievski, A., Mitevska, I., Srbinovska Kostovska, E. Predictors for prognosis in patients with nonfatal Pulmonary Embolism: A Registry-Based Cohort Study. *Clinical and Applied Thrombosis/Hemostasis*. 2018: Vol. 24(95)845-885.

Bossone, E, D'Andrea, A., D'Alto, M., Citro, R., Argiento, P., Ferrara, F., Cittadini, A., Rubenfire, M., Naeije, R. Echocardiography in Pulmonary arterial Hypertension: from Doagnosis to Prognosis, State of the art review article; *Journal of the American Society of Echocardiography,* Vol. 26, No.1,2013.

Bryce, Y. C., Perez-Johnston, R., Bryce, E. B., Homayoon, B., Santos-Martin, E. G., Pathophysiology of right ventricular failure in acute pulmonary embolism and chronic thromboembolic pulmonary hypertension: a pictorial essay for the interventional radiologist; *Insights into imaging* (2019) 10:18.

Chan, W. S., Rey, E., Kent, N. E. VTE in Pregnancy Guideline Working Group; Wee-Shian Chan WS, Kent NE, Rey E, Corbett T, David M, Douglas MJ, Gibson PS, Magee L, Rodger M, Smith RE; Society of Obstetricians and Gynecologists of Canada. Venous thromboembolism and antithrombotic therapy in pregnancy. *J. Obstet Gynaecol Can.* 2014;36(6):527-553.

Cho, J. H., Sridharan, G. K., Kim, H. S., Kaw, R., Abburi, T., Irfan, A., Kocheril, A. G. Right ventricular dysfunction as an echocardiographic prognostic factor in hemodynamically stable patients with acute pulmonary embolism: a meta-analysis; *BMC Cardiovasc Disord.* 2014 May 6; 14:64.

Cohen, R., Loarte, P., Navarro, V., Mirrer, B. Echocardiographic findings in pulmonary embolism: An important guide for the management of the patient; *World Journal of Cardiovascular Diseases*, Vol. 2 No. 3 (2012).

Dabbouseh, N. M, Patel, J. J., Bergel, P. A.: Role of echocardiography in managing acute pulmonary embolism. *Heart*. 2019:105(23):1785-1792.

Dahhan, T., Siddiqui, I., Tapson, V. F., Velazquez, E. J., Sun, S., Davenport, C. A., Samad, Z., Rajagopal, S. Clinical and echocardiographic predictors of mortality in acute pulmonary embolism. *Cardiovasc Ultrasound*. 2016;14 (1):44.

Farag, A., Fielding, J., Catanzano, T., Role of dual energy computed tomography in diagnosis of acute pulmonary emboli, a review. *Semin. Ultr asound* CT MR. 2022; 43(4):333-343.

Hockstein, M. A., Haycock, K., Wiepking, M. Lentz, S., Dugar, S., Siuba, M.: Transthoracic right heart echocardiography for intensivist. *J. Intensive Care Med*, 2021; 36(9):1098-1109.

Humbert, M., Kovacs, G., Hoeper, M. M., Badagliacca, R., Berger, R. M., Brida, M., Carlsen, J., Coats, A. J., Escribano-Subias, P., Ferrari, P., Ferreira, D. S., Ghofrani, H. A., Giannakoulas, G., Kiely, D. G., Mayer, E., Meszaros, G., Nagavci, B., Olsson, K. M., Pepke-Zaba, J., Quint, J. K., Rådegran, G., Simonneau, G., Sitbon, O., Tonia, T., Toshner, M., Vachiery, J. L., Noordegraaf, A. V., Delcroix, M., Rosenkranz, S. the ESC/ERS Scientific Document Group. 2022 ESC/ERS Guidelines for diagnosis and treatment of pulmonary hypertension; *Eur Respir J.* 2023 Jan 6;61(1):2200879.

Jones, N., Burns, A. T., Prior, D.: Echocardiographic Assessment of the Right Ventricle–State of the Art; *Heart, Lung and Circulation* (2019) 28, 1339–1350.

Kim, H. Y., Kim, K. H., Park, J. C.: Multimodality cardiovascular Imaging in pulmonary embolism, *Cardiology Journal* (2021) Vol. 26, No.1,150-160.

Konstantinides, S. V., Meyer, G., Becattini, C., Bueno, H., Geersing, G. J., Harjola, V. P., Huisman, M. V., Humbert, M., Jennings, C. S., Jiménez, D., Kucher, N., Lang, I. M., Lankeit, M., Lorusso, R., Mazzolai, L, Meneveau, N., Áinle, F. N, Prandoni, P., Pruszczyk, P., Righini, M., Torbicki, A., Belle, E. V., Zamorano, J. L., ESC Scientific Document Group. ESC Guidelines for the diagnosis and management of acute pulmonary embolism developed in collaboration with the European Respiratory Society (ERS). *Eur Heart J.* 2020 Jan 21;41(4):543-603.

Konstantinides, S. V., Torbicki, A., Agnelli, G., Danchin, N., Fitzmaurice, D., Galiè, N., Gibbs, J. S., Huisman M. V., Humbert, M., Kucher, N., Lang, I., Lankeit, M., Lekakis, J., Maack, C., Mayer E., Meneveau, N., Perrier, A., Pruszczyk, P., Rasmussen, L. H., Schindler, T. H., Svitil, P., Noordegraaf, A. V., Zamorano, J. L., Zompatori, M. 2014 ESC Guidelines on the diagnosis and management of acute pulmonary embolism: The Task Force for the Diagnosis and Management of Acute Pulmonary Embolism of the European Society of Cardiology (ESC, Endorsed by the European Respiratory Society (ERS); *European Heart Journal*, (2014)35,3033–3080.

Kucher, N., Rossi, E, De Rosa, M., Goldhaber, S. Z. Prognostic role of echocardiography among patients with acute pulmonary embolism and a systolic arterial pressure of 90 mm Hg or higher. *Arch Intern Med.* 2005;165(15):1777–1781.

Lang, R. M., Badano, L., Mor-Avi, V., Afilalo, J., Armstrong, A., Ernande, L., Flachskampf, F. A., Foster, E., Goldstein, S.A., Kuznetsova, T., Lancellotti, P., Muraru, D., Picard, M.H., Rietzschel, E.R., Rudski, L., Spencer, K.T., Tsang, W., Voigt, J. U. Recommendations for Cardiac Chamber Quantification by Echocardiography in Adults: An Update from the American Society of Echocardiography and the European Association of Cardiovascular Imaging; *J Am Soc Echocardiogr.* Volume 28 Number 1, 2015.

Lee, J. H. and Park, J. H., Role of Echocardiography in Patients With Acute Pulmonary Thromboembolism; *J Cardiovasc Ultrasound.* 2008 Mar;16(1):9-16.

Lopez-Candales, A., Dohi, K., Rajagopalan, N., Edelman, K., Gulyasy, B., Bazaz, R. Defining normal variables of right ventricular size and function in pulmonary hypertension: an echocardiographic study. *Postgrad Med J.* 2008; 84:40-5.

Mc Connell, M. V., Solomon, S. D., Rayan, M. E., Come, P. C., Goldhaber, S. Z., Lee, R. T.. Regional right ventricular dysfunction detected by echocardiography in acute pulmonary embolism. *Am J Cardiol.* 1996;78(4):469–473.

McDonagh, T. A., Metra, M., Adamo, M., Gardner, R. S., Baumbach, A., Böhm, M., Burri, H., Butler, J., Čelutkienė, J,, Chioncel, O., Cleland, J. G., Coats, A. J., Crespo-Leiro, M. G., Farmakis, D., Gilard, M., Heymans, S., Hoes, A. W., Jaarsma, T., Jankowska, E. A., Lainscak, M., Lam, C. S., Lyon, A. R., McMurray, J. J., Mebazaa, A., Mindham, R., Muneretto, C., Piepoli, M. F., Price, S., Rosano, G. M., Ruschitzka, F., Skibelund, A. K., ESC Scientific Document Group. 2021 ESC Guidelines for the diagnosis and treatment of acute and chronic heart failure. Developed by the Task Force for the diagnosis and treatment of acute and chronic heart failure of the European Society of Cardiology (ESC) with the special contribution of the Heart Failure Association (HFA) of the ESC; *Eur Heart J* (2021) 42, 3599-3726.

Morris, T. A., Fernandes, T. M., Channick, R.: How we do it: evaluation of dyspnea and exercise intolerance after acute pulmonary embolism. *Chest. Open* Access, July 2, 2022.

Nazerian, P., Gigli, Ch., Reissig, A., Pivetta, E., Vanni, S., Fraccalini, T., Ferraris, G., Ricciardolo A., Grifoni, S., Volpicelli, G; WINFOCUS and US SIMEU study group. Retrospective analysis of the diagnostic accuracy of lung ultrasound for pulmonary embolism in patients with and without pleuritic chest pain; *The Ultrasound Journal volume 14*, Article number: 35 (2022).

Oh, J. K., Park, J. K.: Role of echocardiography in acute pulmonary embolism; 2023. *The KJIM*, 2023, Jan.2.

Pleszewski, B., Chartrand-Lefebvre, C., Qanadil, S. D., Dery, R., Perreault, P., Oliva, V. L., Prenovault, J., Belblidia, A., Soulez, G. Gadolinium enhanced pulmonary magnetic resonance angiography in the diagnosis of acute pulmonary embolism: a prospective study on 48 patients. *Clin. Imaging*. 2006; 30(3):166-172.

Poor, H., Serrao, G., Grapsa, J., Chandrashekhar, Y. S., Bianco, A., Lookstein, R. A., Fuster, V. High risk pulmonary embolism during labor; JACC Case reports; (2023) Vol. 6: 1-9.

Qanadli, S. D., Hajjam, M. E., Vieillard-Baron, A., Joseph, T., Mesurolle, T. B., Oliva, V. L., Barré, O., Bruckert, F., Dubourg, O., Lacombe, O.P. New CT index to quantify arterial obstruction in pulmonary embolism: comparison with angiographic index and echocardiography. *AJR Am J Roentgenol*.2001;176(6):1415-1420.

Quintero-Martinez, J. A., Wysokinski, W. E., Cordova-Madera, S. N., Mogollon, R. J., Garcia-Arango, M., Vlazny, D. T., Houghton, D. E., Casanegra A. I., Villarraga, H. R. Pulmonary artery capacitance and pulmonary vascular resistance as prognostic indicator in acute pulmonary embolism. *Eur Heart J*. Open. 2022:2(2): oeac 007.

Rudski, L. G., Lai, W. W., Afilalo, J., Hua, L., Handschumacher, M. D., Chandrasekaran, K., Solomon, S. D., Louie, E. K., Schiller, N. B. Guidelines for the Echocardiographic Assessment of the Right Heart in Adults: A Report from the American Society of Echocardiography Endorsed by the European Association of Echocardiography, a registered branch of the European Society of Cardiology, and the Canadian Society of Echocardiography; *J Am Soc Echocardiogr* 2010;23:685-713.

Schoepf, U. J., Kucher, N., Kipfmueller, F., Quiroz, R., Costello, P., Goldhaber, S. Z.: Right ventricular enlargement on chest computed tomography: a predictor of early death in acute pulmonary embolism. *Circulation* 2004; 110 (20):3276-3280.

Seon, H. J., Kim, K. H., Lee, W. S., Choi, S., Yoon, H. J., Ahn, Y., Kim, Y. H., Jeong, M. H., Cho, J. G., Park, J. C., Kang, J. C. Usefulness of computed tomography pulmonary angiography in the risk stratification of acute pulmonary thromboembolism. Comparison with cardiac biomarkers. *Circ. J*. 2011; 75(2):428-436.

Srbinovska Kostovska, E.: Role of echocardiography in diagnosis of pulmonary hypertension; *Cardiol Croat*. 2013;8(7-8):258-263.

Stein, P. D., Fowler, S. E., Goodman, L. R., Gottschalk, A., Hales, C. A., Hull, R. D., Leeper, K. V., Popovich, J. A, Quinn, D. A., Sos, T. A., Sostman, H. D., Tapson, V. F., Wakefield, T. W., Weg, J. G., Woodard, P. K., PIOPED II Investigators. Multidetector computed tomography for acute pulmonary embolism. *N. Engl. J. Med*. (2006);354(22):2317-2337.

Squizzato, A., Galli, L. and Gerdes, V. E. A.: Point-of-care ultrasound in the diagnosis of pulmonary embolism; *Critical Ultrasound Journal,* volume 7, Article number: 7 (2015).

Vamsidhar, A., Rajasekhar, D., Vanajakshamma, V., Lakshmi, A. Y., Latheef, K., Sankara, C. S., Reddy, G. O. Comparison of PESI, echocardiogram, CTPA, and NT-proBNP as risk stratification tools in patients with acute pulmonary embolism. *Indian Heart J*. 2017;69(1):68-74.

Vedovati, M. C., Germini, F., Angelli, G., Becattini, C. Prognostic role of embolic burden assessed at computed tomography angiography in patients with acute pulmonary embolism: systematic review and meta-analysis. *J. Thromb Haemost.* 2013;11(12):2092-2102.

Wan, T., Skeith, L., Karovitch, A., Rodger, M., Le Gal G. Guidance for the diagnosis of pulmonary embolism during pregnancy: Consensus and controversies. *Thromb Res.* 2017; 157:23-28.

Zaidi, A., Knight, D. S., Augustine, D. X., Harkness, A., Oxborough, D., Pearce, P., Ring, L., Robinson, S., Stout, M., Willis, J., Sharma, V., and the Education Committee of the British Society of Echocardiography: Echocardiographic assessment of the right heart in adults: a practical guideline from the British Society of Echocardiography; *Echo Res Pract.* 2020 Mar; 7(1): G19–G41.

Zhu, R., and Xiao-Chun, M.: Clinical Value of Ultrasonography in Diagnosis of Pulmonary Embolism in Critically Ill Patients; *J Transl Int Med.* 2017 Dec; 5(4): 200–204.

Chapter 5

Medical Treatment of Acute Pulmonary Thromboembolism

Irena Mitevska*, PhD

University Cardiology Clinic, Clinical Center, Medical Faculty, Saints Cyril and Metodij University Skopje, North Macedonia

Abstract

The individual treatment approach in patients with acute pulmonary embolism (PE) is of great importance for patients' intra-hospital outcomes and prognosis. It is one of the key elements of the pulmonary embolism circle of clinical care, strictly described in the several latest PE guidelines from many medical societies. Treatment decisions are guided by patients' assessed risk. Patients with acute PE are at high risk for death, PE recurrence, or development of chronic thromboembolic pulmonary hypertension. Appropriate and fast treatment can potentially reduce the incidence of all PE complications. PE mortality can be up to 30% in undiagnosed and untreated individuals, which is over 10 times higher than the annual mortality in patients treated with anticoagulant therapy (approximately 2.5%). Additionally, the balance between the choice of anticoagulant therapy and bleeding risk should always be assessed. Therapeutic decisions for acute PE have been investigated for decades, with many rapid advances in medical, invasive, and surgical approaches. Currently available management strategies involve systemic fibrinolysis, anticoagulation therapy with unfractionated heparin (UH), low molecular weight heparin (LMWH), direct oral anticoagulant drugs (DOACs), vitamin K antagonists (VKA), catheter-based fibrinolysis, catheter and surgical pulmonary embolectomy, and vena cava filters. This chapter describes medical treatment choices in patients with acute PE.

* Corresponding Author's Email: peovskai@yahoo.com.

In: Pulmonary Embolism
Editors: Irena Mitevska, Sonja Salinger, Marijan Bosevski et al.
ISBN: 979-8-89113-175-0

Keywords: pulmonary embolism, thrombolysis, anticoagulation therapy, direct oral anticoagulation drugs

Introduction

Patients with PE have a higher risk for death, PE recurrence, and increased long-term morbidity. With appropriate treatment, we can reduce the incidence of all potential complications. PE mortality in untreated patients is up to 30%, over 10 times higher than the annual mortality for patients treated with anticoagulants (2.5%) (Bělohlávek et al., 2013). The long-term sequelae of acute PE significantly burden the patients and the health care system. Once the diagnosis of PE is confirmed, it is critical to initiate treatment immediately since it is an emergency medical condition. Anticoagulation therapies include heparin, warfarin, and direct oral anticoagulants (DOACs), with major developments in the last decade. The introduction of DOACs as revolutionary anticoagulant therapy for PE provides simple and safe therapy in broad patient profiles. DOACs reduced bleeding complications and PE recurrence rate, which reflects in reduced mortality. Anticoagulation therapy inhibits certain aspects of the hemostasis system to prevent thrombus growth and propagation. It is critical to monitor for signs and symptoms of bleeding, food, and drug interactions, as well as therapy efficacy associated with improved patient outcomes. Another modality of therapy includes fibrinolysis, catheter-directed therapies, and surgical embolectomy used in high-risk unstable patients (Kasper et al., 1997). Inferior vena cava (IVC) filter insertion can be used in patients with contraindications to anticoagulation, anticoagulant-induced hypercoagulation, or patients with high bleeding risk (Wassef et al., 2017).

Selection of Anticoagulants and Treatment Modalities for Pulmonary Embolism

The General Principle of Anticoagulation

The goal of acute pulmonary embolism (PE) treatment is to prevent thrombus extension and embolization, protect lung circulation, and reduce mortality. Long-term therapeutic goals are reduction of the risk of recurrent pulmonary embolism, development of chronic thromboembolic pulmonary hypertension

(CTEPH) and improvement of the patient's quality of life. Medical anticoagulation therapy consists of three phases: acute phase (the first 5–21 days), long-term phase (3–6 months), and extended phase (after the sixth month, as shown in Figure 1). In the acute period, the main anticoagulation therapy is heparin-based or oral anticoagulant therapy in stable patients and systemic or catheter fibrinolytic therapy, catheter or surgical pulmonary embolectomy in high-risk clinically unstable patients. For long-term treatment, the general anticoagulant treatment period for provoked PE is three months because of the low risk of recurrence, and up to six months in patients with unprovoked PE (Konstantinides et al., 2020). Extended treatment can be considered in patients with a high risk of recurrent PE episodes. DOACs are preferred drugs for long-term and extended treatment, excluding patients with severe mitral valve stenosis or mechanical mitral valve, antiphospholipid syndrome, pregnancy, and breast feeding, as well as severe renal and liver failure.

Pulmonary Embolism Treatment in High Risk Patients

Hemodynamic and Respiratory Support in High-Risk Pulmonary Embolism

High-risk patients represent 5% of all PE cases with high intra-hospital mortality. Hypoxemia is commonly present in cases with massive high-risk PE, mostly caused by the mismatch between ventilation and perfusion. Administration of supplemental oxygen is indicated in patients with PE and reduced oxygen saturation (SaO2) < 90%. In the presence of severe respiratory failure, high-flow oxygen and mechanical ventilation (non-invasive or invasive) should be applied. Mechanical ventilation, however, may cause further hemodynamic deterioration by decreasing the venous return. In the case of reduced cardiac output, the dilated and dysfunctional right ventricle is unlikely to respond to inotropic agents, which may provoke arrhythmias (Konstantinides et al., 2020). When necessary, or in the presence of shock, cautious use of noradrenaline might be beneficial for improving right ventricular function and systemic hemodynamics. Based on the smaller studies results, the use of dobutamine may be considered for patients with PE, low cardiac index, and normal blood pressure, bearing in mind that raising the cardiac index may worsen ventilation/perfusion mismatch. Although experimental data suggest that levosimendan causes pulmonary vasodilation with an increase in *right ventricular* (RV) contractility, there are no significant evidences of clinical benefits (Hansen et al., 2018). Fluid loading might be dangerous in case of sudden RV dilatation and high filling pressure, which can further shift inter-ventricular septum leftward, and can further cause a decrease in left ventricular output. Vasodilators should be generally avoided in the setting of high-risk acute PE (Konstantinides et al., 2020)). Assessment of central venous pressure by ultrasound imaging of the inferior vena cava or by central venous pressure monitoring may help guide volume loading. The temporary use of mechanical cardiopulmonary support, usually with veno-arterial extracorporeal membrane oxygenation (ECMO), may be helpful in patients with high-risk PE with obstructive shock or cardiac resuscitation. However, there are no larger randomized trials assessing the efficacy and safety of these devices in high-risk PE. Use of ECMO is associated with a high incidence of complications, and results depend on the center experience and appropriate patient selection (Stevens et al., 2021).

Thrombolytic Therapy

Systemic thrombolysis is a treatment of choice in high-risk hemodynamically unstable patients, as defined in Chapter 1 of this book (Class IA). Thrombolytic treatment, by actively dissolving the clot, can quickly reduce the load on the right ventricle and has the potential to prevent death in the hemodynamically unstable patient. The recommended fibrinolytic medications and appropriate dosage are available in the current PE guideline (Table 1). Intermediate high-risk patients are the most challenging group where sudden clinical deterioration might happen. The latest European Society of Cardiology (ESC) classification of PE patients has an insufficient positive predictive value to identify a subgroup of intermediate-risk patients who might need more aggressive therapy. The benefits of full-dose systemic thrombolysis are outweighed by bleeding risks. However, identification of higher-risk patients and improvement of the safety of thrombolytic therapy might improve the risk-benefit ratio of this therapy in intermediate-risk patients (Meyer et al. 2014, Sharifi et al., 2013). It remains unclear whether early thrombolysis in these patients has an impact on clinical symptoms, functional status, or CTEPH at long-term follow up. A small randomized trial suggested that thrombolysis might improve functional capacity at three months compared with anticoagulation alone. The pulmonary embolism thrombolysis (PEITHO) trial results do not support a role for thrombolysis in preventing long-term sequelae in intermediate-risk PE, although clinical follow-up was available in only 62% of the evaluated population (Mayer et al., 2014; Chatterjee et al., 2014). There are research trials assessing the effectiveness of half-dose rtPA or dose adjuster protocol (0.6 mg/kg) in intermediate high-risk patients (Teleb et al., 2016; Taherkhani et al., 2014). The ongoing PEITHO-3 trial is expected to give an answer and position of the thrombolytic therapy in intermediate-high-risk patients. The results from the Regional Pulmonary Embolism Registry (REPER) showed that slow low-dose rtPA, (1–5 mg/h, maximum dose 20–50 mg) applied either by intravenous or by local catheter infusion, resulted in reduced hospital mortality compared to classic faster, high-dose rtPA protocols in the intermediate-high-risk patients (Obradovic et al., Srce i Krvni Sudovi, 2022).

The most frequently used parameters of the therapeutic effectiveness of thrombolytic therapy are clinical hemodynamic improvement and degree of angiographic or scintigraphic thrombus resolution. Systemic thrombolysis induces faster early resolution of pulmonary embolus than unfractionated heparin (UFH); however, no significant difference was found after several days. An additional factor contributing to the lack of significant reduction of mortality despite impressive early thrombus resolution is that patients who survive long enough to be entered into a clinical trial probably make up a group with an improved prognosis, and the most unstable high-risk patients will probably die before receiving proper treatment. The rate of treatment failure in high-risk patients is lower in those treated with thrombolytics than in those who receive UFH. Further indirect evidence comes from a multicenter registry in patients without shock, where in patients treated with thrombolysis, 30-day mortality was significantly lower (4.7% *vs.* 11.1%) with significantly less recurrent pulmonary embolism (7.7% *vs.* 18.7%) compared to the group treated with heparin (Nagamalesh et al., 2017). Additional meta-analysis showed that the use of thrombolytics was associated with lower all-cause mortality, mainly in studies including hemodynamically unstable patients (Chatterjee et al., 2014). In a large North American database that includes over two million patients with PE, intra-hospital mortality was 15% among patients with unstable PE receiving thrombolytic therapy and 47% among patients with unstable PE treated with anticoagulant therapy alone (Douketis et al., 1998). Management decisions based on the patient's risk stratification and hemodynamic stability are shown in Figure 1.

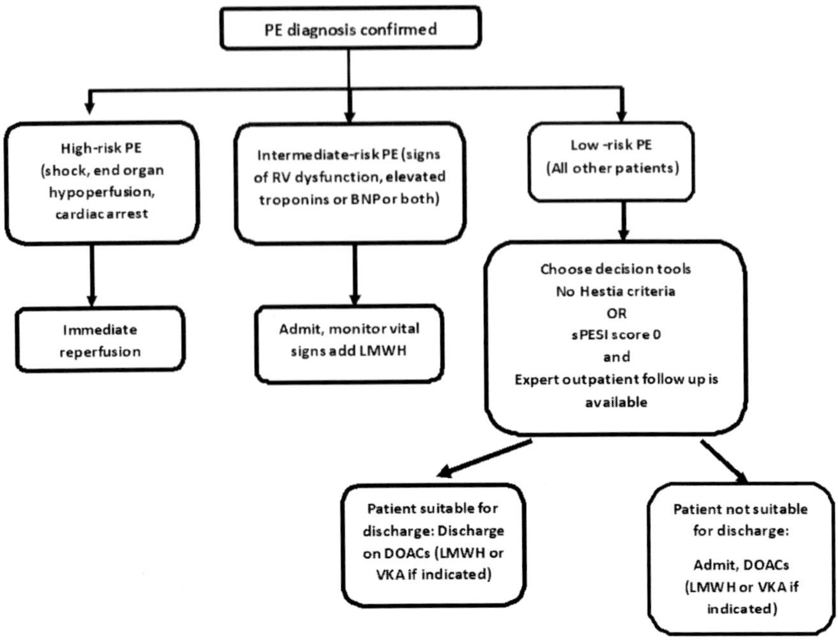

PE- pulmonary embolism; LMWH- low molecular weight heparin; DOACs- direct oral anticoagulant therapy, sPESI- simplified pulmonary embolism severity index; VKA- vitamin K antagonists.

Figure 1. Pulmonary Embolism treatment approach based on patient risk stratification.

Contrary to the patients with acute myocardial infarction, thrombolysis in acute PE is effective for 10–14 days after the onset of symptoms. Generally accepted dosing recommendations and fibrinolysis contraindications are given in Table 1. There is no need to obtain clotting tests during fibrinolytic treatment as those tests will not predict eventual complications or adjust the drug dose. After the thrombolytic treatment, measurements of activated partial thromboplastin clotting time (aPTT) and fibrinogen are mandatory in order to determine when heparin therapy should be applied. If the post-thrombolysis aPTT values exceed twice the upper limit of normal or the fibrinogen concentration is below 1 g/l, the tests should be repeated every four hours until they reach concentrations, at which point heparin can be started (or resumed) safely (Wang et al., 2010; Kearon et al., 2008). The main complication of thrombolytic treatment is bleeding. The average overall major hemorrhage incidence with thrombolysis in PE is approximately 10% and is similar among used thrombolytic agents. The bleeding risk is increased in elderly patients with uncontrolled hypertension and those with recent stroke or brain surgery.

Table 1. Thrombolythic drugs, dosing, and contraindications

Fibrinolytic drug	Dosing regimen	Contraindications to fibrinolysis
rtPA	100 mg over 2 h 0.6 mg/kg over 15 min (maximum dose 50 mg)	Absolute History of bleeding, stroke of unknown origin Ischemic stroke in the last 6 months Central nervous system cancer Major trauma, surgery, head injury in the last 3 months Bleeding diathesis Active bleeding Relative Transient ischemic attack in the last 6 months Oral anticoagulation Pregnancy or fist postpartum week Non-compression puncture sites Traumatic resuscitation Refractory hypertension Advanced liver disease Infective endocarditis Active peptic ulcer
Streptokinase	250.000 IU as loading dose over 30 min, followed by 100.000 IU/h over 12-24 h Accelerated regimen: 1.5 mil IU over 2 h	
Urokinase	4400 IU/kg as loading dose over 10 minutes followed by 4400 IU kg/h over 12-24 h Accelerated regimen: 3 mil IU over 2 h	

rtPA- recombinant tissue plasminogen activator.

Anticoagulation Therapy for Acute Pulmonary Embolism

The initial treatment of hemodynamically stable patients with pulmonary embolism (PE) has dramatically changed since the introduction of low molecular weight heparins (LMWHs). With the inclusion of the DOACs, the initial treatment of PE is further simplified, more secure, and non-inferior to the treatment with LMWH (Kahn et al., 2022). The practical use of DOACs place them as agents of first choice in the initial treatment of stable PE patients (Kakkos et al., 2014; Witt et al., 2018; National Institute for Health and Care Excellence, 2020).

Treatment of Intermediate High-Risk Patients

Unfractionated Heparin Therapy

In patients with high or intermediate PE probability (Chapter 1), anticoagulation should be initiated while waiting for the results of ongoing diagnostic tests. For this purpose, we can use weight-adjusted low-molecular-weight heparin (LMWH) or fondaparinux, or intravenous unfractionated heparin (UFH) (Buller et al., 2003). Close monitoring is necessary for these patient populations, since hemodynamic deterioration, even in the first five days from diagnosis, is possible, where a switch to thrombolytic therapy might be necessary. LMWH and fondaparinux are recommended over UFH for initial anticoagulation in PE due to lower risk of major bleeding or heparin-induced thrombocytopenia (HIT). Additionally, LMWH and fondaparinux do not need routine monitoring of anti-Xa levels or hemostasis parameters. Use of UFH is mostly restricted to patients with advanced hemodynamic instability, or signs of hemodynamic worsening; primary reperfusion treatment might be used. UFH is also recommended for patients with serious renal impairment (creatinine clearance (CrCl) < 30 mg/ml, dosing adjusted based on the aPTT) (Robertson et al. 2017; Lasica et al., 2022). Based on several expert opinions, after fibrinolytic therapy, the use of UFH should be maintained for the additional 48 hours with close hemodynamic monitoring (Lauren et al., 2020). This is the period of shock recovery, with the presence of potential renal dysfunction. After that period of clinical stabilization, LMWH or NOACs may be introduced.

The efficacy of heparin treatment depends on achieving a critical therapeutic concentration of heparin within the first few hours of treatment. An initial bolus of UFH could be considered since UFH has a rapid onset of action, short half-life, the ability for fast and safer use of thrombolysis, invasive procedures, and easier management of major bleedings (Hirsh et al., 2004). The initial bolus of UFH also overcomes the delay in the onset of full anticoagulation. Preclinical evidence that UFH inhibits platelets serotonin release associated with a decrease in vasospasm and bronchospasm may be of additional clinical value. In all intermediate-risk PE patients, despite the choice of initial therapy, careful monitoring during the first 24 h is recommended, irrespective of the initially used therapy.

Compared to LMWH, UFH has unpredictable pharmacokinetics due to a small volume of distribution and variable half-life, and extensive binding to plasma proteins, which result in a therapeutic range only 22% of the time in the setting of acute PE (Aday AW et al., 2020). Considering UFH dosing, two options were available: standard dosing, which includes a bolus of 80 U/kg followed by an infusion at 18 U/kg/h, or an infusion-only regimen, which consisted of an infusion at 18 U/kg/h without a bolus. Assessment for bleeding risk, renal and liver function is mandatory for each patient. UFH plasma concentrations and anticoagulant response are unpredictable; therefore the aPTT test is advised to be performed 4–6 hours after initiation of the treatment and repeated six hours after any change of dosage, and subsequently at least daily. The aPTT should be maintained at 1.5–2.5 times the patient pretreatment or the laboratory mean referent value. Failure to achieve this range is associated with an increased risk of recurrent venous thromboembolism. In contrast, there is only a weak association between supratherapeutic aPTT response and the risk of bleeding. True heparin resistance is mainly caused by ATIII deficiency.

Heparin therapy in intermediate high-risk and high-risk patients should be applied for 24–36 hours, based on expert opinions and trial results, although these time frames are not precisely described in the latest PE guidelines (Konstantinides et al., 2020). Oral anticoagulants with vitamin K antagonists (VKA) and dabigatran should be started together with heparin treatment, and these should be administered jointly for at least five days. Heparin may be stopped when the international normalized ratio (INR) is above 2.0 on two consecutive days for patients on VKA. Many patients who suffer recurrence while receiving heparin will be found to be inadequately anticoagulated, as reflected by an aPTT below the therapeutic range. Increasing the dose of heparin should be the initial alteration in treatment in these patients. Bleeding complications are reported in up to 15% of patients on full-dose heparin, with less than 5% of major bleedings (Mark et al., 2008). They are most likely if the patient with a pre-existing bleeding tendency, uremia, advanced age, recent surgery or trauma, uncontrolled hypertension, previous gastrointestinal hemorrhage, and concomitant antiplatelet treatment.

UFH causes transient mild thrombocytopenia in approximately 10% of patients and severe thrombocytopenia in less than 5% (Ahmed et al., 2007). The severe heparin-induced thrombocytopenia (HIT) occurs five or more days after starting heparin treatment. In confirmed cases, heparin therapy must be stopped, and recombinant hirudin or bivalirudin should be given for temporary anticoagulation. The use of oral anticoagulants and platelet transfusions in the acute phase of HIT may worsen the thrombotic tendency. All anticoagulant treatment options for acute and long PE phases are shown in Table 2.

Low Molecular Weight Heparin

Low-molecular-weight heparin is the preferred immediate anticoagulant for patients with intermediate-risk pulmonary embolism. It leads to less major bleeding and lower mortality compared to UFH. LMWH dosing of 1 mg/kg in 12-hour intervals should be used. Compared to UFH, LMWH is more likely to show a predictable dose–response relationship, and it does not require routine hemostasis monitoring (Garcia et al., 2012). Factor Xa can be monitored in case of assessing eventual efficacy. It has a longer half-life, allowing it to be administered subcutaneously once or twice a day, with a lower risk of HIT and osteoporosis. Because LMWH is excreted mainly by the kidney, it should not be used in patients with severe renal impairment. The preference for therapeutic use of LMWH or subcutaneous fondaparinux, which have similar beneficial effects and harms, should be guided by clinician experience, costs, and availability.

Oral Anticoagulants

Oral anticoagulation therapy is one of the treatment options in intermediate high- and low-risk patients during the hospital's initial management phase, as well as for long-term anticoagulant treatment. Two groups of drugs, VKA and DOACs, might be used in both treatment phases. Duration of oral anticoagulation should be individually assessed, balancing the bleeding risk and the risk of PE recurrence. Patients with transient major provoking risk factors should be treated for minimum of three months up to six months, assuring there is no persisting risk factor. In patients with unprovoked, recurrent PE, active tumors, thrombophilia, and antiphospholipid syndrome, longer or indefinite anticoagulation therapy is required.

Direct Oral Anticoagulant Therapy

DOACs are medications that revolutionized the treatment of DVT and PE. DOACs have the potential to simplify the management of PE, thanks to unique pharmacologic properties (rapid onset of action, short half-life, and predictable anticoagulant effect), which make them at least as safe and effective as conventional anticoagulant therapy, with lower rates of intracranial bleedings and the absence of routine laboratory monitoring. For all these reasons, DOACs also appear as an attractive treatment strategy for the outpatient management of selected patients with PE. The availability of antidotes in case of bleeding is another advantage (Kakkos et al., 2014). Major phase 3 randomized trials (EINSTEIN, AMPLIFY, RECOVER, and HOKUSAI) showed that DOACs had a similar efficacy and better safety than conventional treatment with parenteral heparin and vitamin K antagonists in acute PE management (Cohen AT et al., 2014). Their predictable bioavailability and pharmacokinetic properties enable them to be fixed in doses without routine laboratory monitoring. Compared with VKA, there are fewer drug and food interactions, improved tolerability, and patient compliance. Apixaban and rivaroxaban can be given in the initial PE treatment phase without previous LMWH treatment. Data from phase III PE trials advise that dosages of dabigatran, rivaroxaban, and apixaban should not be reduced in patients with mild-moderate renal dysfunction (creatinine clearance - CrCl between 30–60 mL/min), whereas edoxaban was given at a 30 mg dose in the same population (Buller HR et al., 2013). DOACs should not be used in patients with advanced renal failure and CrCl below 15 ml/min, during pregnancy and lactation, and in patients with the antiphospholipid antibody syndrome. The latest PE guidelines from several professional associations indicate DOAC as the preferred treatment option in stable PE when oral anticoagulation is used. This is a strong (class I, A) recommendation based on the evidence from large clinical trials which led to the clinical approval of DOACs. Those trials showed treatment non-inferiority and superior safety of NOACs compared to the LMWH and VKA in acute PE treatment. The EINSTEIN-EXTENSION trial confirmed the superior efficacy of rivaroxaban compared to the VKA in the secondary prevention of PE, showing reductions in primary outcome of symptomatic recurrent PE with an acceptable major bleeding rate in the period of 6–12 months of prolonged treatment (Weitz et al, 2017).

Vitamin K Antagonists

Vitamin K antagonists (VKA) have been the historic gold standard for oral anticoagulation in the last 50 years. When VKAs are used, anticoagulation with UFH, LMWH, or fondaparinux should be continued in parallel with the oral anticoagulant for > 5 days and until the international normalized ratio (INR) value has been 2–3 for two consecutive days. There are many pharmacological characteristics of the VKAs that make them insufficient compared to DOACs (variations or anticoagulant activity and a longer period to achieve maximal therapeutic effects, more drug and food interaction, need for monitoring of anticoagulant activity, lower compliance rate).

Table 2. Modalities of anticoagulant therapy in acute pulmonary embolism (modified from Kahn SR, 2022)

Acute period (first 5-21 days)	Long-term period (3 to 6 months)	Extended period (beyond long-term period)
→	→	→
UFH/LMWH (lead minimum 5 days)	Warfarin: target therapeutic level INR 2-3	If required
UFH/LMWH (lead minimum 5 days)	LMWH: in case of CAT therapeutic dose	If required
UFH/LMWH (lead in first 5 days)	aEdoxaban: 60 mg oad (30 mg/day if body weight<60 kg or CrCl 30–50 ml/min)	If required
UFH/LMWH (lead in first 5 days)	aDabigatran: 150 mg twice daily	If required
Rivaroxaban: 15 mg twice daily (first 21 days)	aRivaroxaban: 20 mg one daily	If required: 10 mg once daily
Apixaban: 10 mg twice daily (first 7 days)	aApixaban: 5 mg twice daily	If required: 2.5 mg twice daily

aDoses can be modified based on body weight, organ function or concomitant medications INR- international normalized ratio; LMWH- low molecular weight heparin; UFH- unfractionated heparin, oad-once daily.

Anticoagulation Treatment in Special Populations

Patients with renal failure. The anticoagulant effect of DOACs increases in the presence of renal insufficiency, also the likelihood of bleeding complications because of the main renal excretion of these drugs. DOAC can be safely use in patients with renal failure, cautious in patients with creatinine clearance of < 30 mL/min, especially with edoxaban trial, and should not be used in advanced renal failure with creatinine clearance of <15 mL/min (Lutz et al., 2017). LMWH can be used safely in patients with moderate renal impairment, with once-daily dosing in patients with creatinine clearance <30 ml/min. For dosage adjustment purposes, it is recommended to monitor the activity of anti-Xa level in order to avoid underdosage and obtain optimal therapeutic activity. UFH is recommended for patients with severe renal insufficiency.

Patients with thrombocytopenia. In cases of carcinoma-associated thrombosis (CAT) and thrombocytopenia, LMWH is the preferred anticoagulant because of its shorter half-life and better safety profile than VKA. DOACs may also be considered for these patients. Most trials with DOACs in CAT excluded patients with a platelet count $<50{,}000\times10^9$/l, and there is insufficient data on whether DOACs can replace LMWH in the setting of CAT with significant thrombocytopenia. (Napolitano et al., 2019).

Patients with subsegmental pulmonary embolism. The decision on whether to treat asymptomatic subsegmental PE patients remains challenging since this issue is not supported by many randomized clinical trials (Carrier et al., 2017). Asymptomatic patients without co-existing deep vein thrombosis (DVT) and high-risk characteristics, recurrent or progressive PE (immobilization, active cancer, unprovoked VTE, high bleeding risk) may have undergone serial lower leg DVT screening without anticoagulation. However, if patients are symptomatic, with co-existing DVT, or have high-risk features and low bleeding risk, anticoagulation might be used. In patients with anticoagulation therapy, drug choice, and the treatment duration may follow the treatment strategies recommended for PE in larger pulmonary arteries. The latest American College of Chest Physicians VTE guidelines recommend subsegmental PE treatment based on individual patient VTE recurrence risk (whether the risk is low or high). In either case, anticoagulation treatment is advised (Stevens et al., 2021).

Patients with incidental pulmonary embolism. Incidental PE is not a rare report on chest CT scans. Although the embolic load is usually lower than that in symptomatic PE, anticoagulation should be used in cases with proximal and subsegmental locations.

Patients with initial anticoagulation treatment failure. The most frequent causes of PE treatment failure and PE recurrence is inadequate anticoagulation therapy (lower dosage, poor compliance, therapy malabsorption, malignancy, inherited thrombophilia, and antiphospholipid antibody syndrome). Treatment options for initial failure include increasing the dose or administration frequency of the anticoagulants or the use of alternate medication. In patients receiving VKA (with an INR of 2.0 to 3.0) or an adequate dose of a DOAC, the guidelines recommend changing to LMWH (Kazmi et al., 2011). In patients receiving LMWH, increasing the LMWH dose by 25 to 33% should be applied. The efficacy of DOACs in this population has not yet been studied.

Conclusion

The management decisions in acute PE require an individual approach and guidelines-based risk stratification. The presence of hemodynamic instability which implies high patient risk, indicated the need for systemic thrombolytic therapy, catheter thrombolysis, and catheter or surgical embolectomy. Low-risk patients can have safe early hospital discharge and be treated as outpatients at home. The intermediate-risk group is a highly heterogeneous group of patients, mostly with favorable short-term outcomes. These patients might be treated with LMWH or directly with DOACs, especially intermediate low-risk patients. Individual evaluations by dedicated multidisciplinary PE teams are useful for deciding the optimal treatment strategy.

References

Aday, A. W. and Beckman, J. A. Pulmonary Embolism and Unfractionated Heparin: Time to End the Roller Coaster Ride. *Acad. Emerg. Med.* 2020 Feb; 27(2): 176–178.

Ahmed, I., Majeed, A., and Powell, R. Heparin induced thrombocytopenia: diagnosis and management update. *Postgrad Med J.* 2007 Sep; 83(983): 575–582.

Bělohlávek, J., Dytrych, V., and Linhart, A. Pulmonary embolism, part I: Epidemiology, risk factors and risk stratification, pathophysiology, clinical presentation, diagnosis and nonthrombotic pulmonary embolism. *Exp. Clin. Cardiol.* 2013;18(2): 129–138.

Büller, H. R., Davidson, B. L., Decousus, H., Gallus, A., Gent, M., Piovella, F., Prins, M. H., Raskob, G., van den Berg-Segers, A. E., Cariou, R., Leeuwenkamp, O., Lensing, A. W.; Matisse Investigators. Subcutaneous fondaparinux versus intravenous unfractionated heparin in the initial treatment of pulmonary embolism. *N. Engl. J. Med.* 2003;349: 1695-1702.

Buller, H. R., Decousus, H., Grosso, M. A., Mercuri, M., Middeldorp, S., Prins, M. H., Raskob, G. E., Schellong, S. M., Schwocho, L., Segers, A., Shi, M., Verhamme, P., Wells, P. Edoxaban versus warfarin for the treatment of symptomatic venous thromboembolism. *N. Engl. J. Med.* 2013; 369:1406-1415.

Carrier, M. and Klok, F. A. Symptomatic subsegmental pulmonary embolism: to treat or not to treat? *Hematology Am Soc Hematol Educ Program.* 2017 Dec 8; 2017(1): 237–241.

Chatterjee, S., Chakraborty, A., Weinberg, I., Kadakia, M., Wilensky, R.L., Sardar, P., Kumbhani, D. J., Mukherjee, D, Jaff, M. R., Giri, J. Thrombolysis for pulmonary embolism and risk of all-cause mortality, major bleeding, and intracranial hemorrhage: a meta-analysis. *JAMA* 2014; 311:2414-21.

Cohen, A.T., Imfeld, S., and Rider, T. Phase III Trials of New Oral Anticoagulants in the Acute Treatment and Secondary Prevention of VTE: Comparison and Critique of Study Methodology and Results. *Adv. Ther.* 2014; 31(5): 473–493.

Douketis, J. D., Kearon, C., Bates, S., Duku, E. K., Ginsberg, J.S. Risk of fatal pulmonary embolism in patients with treated venous thromboembolism. *JAMA*. 1998 Feb 11;279(6):458-62.

Garcia, D. A., Baglin, T. P., Weitz, J. I. and Samama, S. Antithrombotic Therapy and Prevention of Thrombosis, 9th ed: American College of Chest Physicians Evidence-Based Clinical Practice Guidelines. *Chest.* 2012 Feb; 141(2 Suppl): e24S–e43S.

Hansen, M. S., Andersen, A., and Nielsen-Kudsk, J. E. Levosimendan in pulmonary hypertension and right heart failure. *Pulm. Circ.* 2018 Jul-Sep; 8(3): 2045894018 790905.

Hirsh, J., Raschke. R. Heparin and low-molecular-weight heparin: the seventh accp conference on antithrombotic and thrombolytic therapy. *Chest.* 2004; 126: 188-203.

Kahn, S. R., and de Wit, K. Pulmonary Embolism. *N. Engl. J. Med.* 2022; 387:45-57.

Kakkos, S. K., Kirkilesis, G. I., Tsolakis, I. A. Editor's Choice - efficacy and safety of the new oral anticoagulant's dabigatran, rivaroxaban, apixaban, and edoxaban in the treatment and secondary prevention of venous thromboembolism: a systematic review and meta-analysis of phase III trials. *Eur. J. Vasc. Endovasc. Surg.* 2014; 48:565-575.

Kasper, W., Konstantinides, S., Geibel, A., Olschewski, M., Heinrich, F., Grosser, K.D., Rauber, K., Iversen, S., Redecker, M., Kienast, J. Management strategies and determinants of outcome in acute major pulmonary embolism: results of a multicenter registry. *J. Am. Coll. Cardiol.* 1997; Vol.30, No.5, p. 1165-71.

Kazmi, R. S. and Lwaleed, B. A. New anticoagulants: how to deal with treatment failure and bleeding complications. *Br. J. Clin. Pharmacol*. 2011 Oct; 72(4): 593–603.

Kearon, C., Kahn, S. R., Agnelli, G., Goldhaber, S., Raskob, G.E. and Comerota, A. J. Antithrombotic therapy for venous thromboembolic disease: American College of Chest Physicians Evidence-Based Clinical Practice Guidelines (8th Edition). *Chest,* 2008; Vol.133, No.6 Suppl, 454S-545S.

Konstantinides, S. V., Meyer, G., Becattini, C., Bueno, H., Geersing, G. J., Harjola, V. P., Huisman, M. V., Humbert, M., Jennings, C. S., Jiménez, D., Kucher, N., Lang, I. M., Lankeit, M., Lorusso, R., Mazzolai, L, Meneveau, N., Áinle, F. N, Prandoni, P., Pruszczyk, P., Righini, M., Torbicki, A., Belle, E.V., Zamorano, J. L.; ESC

Scientific Document Group. ESC Guidelines for the diagnosis and management of acute pulmonary embolism developed in collaboration with the European Respiratory Society (ERS). *Eur. Heart J.* 2020 Jan 21;41(4):543-603.

Lasica, R., Asanin, M., Djukanovic, L., Radovanovic, N., Savic, L., Polovina, M. Stankovic, S., Ristic, A., Zdravkovic, M., Lasica,. A., Kravic, J., Perunic, J. Dilemmas in the Choice of Adequate Therapeutic Treatment in Patients with Acute Pulmonary Embolism-From Modern Recommendations to Clinical Application. *Pharmaceuticals* (Basel). 2022 Sep; 15(9): 1146.

Stewart, L.K, Kline, J.A. Fibrinolytics for the treatment of pulmonary embolism. *Transl. Res.* 2020 Nov; 225: 82–94.

Lutz. J, Jurk. K, and Schinzel, H. Direct oral anticoagulants in patients with chronic kidney disease: patient selection and special considerations. *Int. J. Nephrol. Renovasc. Dis.* 2017; 10: 135–143.

Crowther, M. A., Warkentin, T. E. Bleeding risk and the management of bleeding complications in patients undergoing anticoagulant therapy: focus on new anticoagulant agents. *Blood* (2008) 111 (10): 4871–4879.

Meyer, G., Vicaut, E., Danays, T., Agnelli, G., Becattini, C., Beyer-Westendorf, J., Bluhmki, E., Bouvaist, H., Brenner, B., Couturaud, F., Dellas, C., Empen, K., Franca, A., Galiè, N., Geibel, A., Goldhaber, S. Z., Jimenez, D., Kozak, M., Kupatt, C., Kucher, N., Lang, I. M., Lankeit, M., Meneveau, N., Pacouret, G., Palazzini, M., Petris, A., Pruszczyk, P., Rugolotto, M., Salvi, A., Schellong, S., Sebbane, M., Sobkowicz, B., Stefanovic, B.S., Thiele, H., Torbicki, A., Verschuren, F., Konstantinides, S.V.; PEITHO Investigators. Fibrinolysis for patients with intermediate risk pulmonary embolism. *N. Eng.l J. Med. 2014*; 370:1402-11.

Nagamalesh, U. M., Prakash, V. S., Naidu, K. C., Sarthak, S., Hegde, A.V., and Abhinay, T. Acute pulmonary thromboembolism: Epidemiology, predictors, and long-term outcome – A single center experience. *Indian Heart J.* 2017 Mar-Apr; 69(2): 160–164.

Napolitano, M., Saccullo, S., Marietta, M., Carpenedo, M., Castaman, M.G., Cerchiara, E., Chistolini, A., Contino, L., De Stefano, V., Falanga, A., Federici, A.B., Rossi, E., Santoro, R., Siragusa, S., and Gruppo Italiano Malattie EMatologiche dell'Adulto (GIMEMA) Working Party on Thrombosis and Hemostasis, on behalf of the *Grupp.* Platelet cut-off for anticoagulant therapy in thrombocytopenic patients with blood cancer and venous thromboembolism: an expert consensus. *Blood Transfus.* 2019 May; 17(3): 171–180.

Obradovic, S. D., Djuric, I. R., Dzudovic, B. M., Subotic, B. N., Dzudovic, J. M., Matijasevic, J.A. What we have learned from the Regional Pulmonary Embolism Registry (REPER)? *Srce i krvni sudovi.* 2022; 41(4): 163-167.

Robertson, L., Jones, L.E. Fixed dose subcutaneous low molecular weight heparins versus adjusted dose unfractionated heparin for the initial treatment of venous thromboembolism. *Cochrane Database Syst Rev* 2017; 2:CD001100.

Sharifi, M., Bay, C., Skrocki, L., Rahimi, F., Mehdipour, M.; MOPETT Investigators. Moderate pulmonary embolism treated with thrombolysis (from the "MOPETT" Trial). *Am. J. Cardiol.* 2013; 111:273-277.

Stevens, S. M., Woller, S. C., Kreuziger, L. B., Bounameaux, H., Doerschug, K., Geersing, G. J., Huisman, M. V., Kearon, C., King, C. S., Knighton, A. J., Lake, E., Murin, S., Vintch, J. R., Wells, P.S., Moores, L. K. Antithrombotic Therapy for VTE Disease: Second Update of the CHEST Guideline and Expert Panel Report. *Chest.* 2021 Dec;160(6): e545-e608.

Taherkhani, M., Taherkhani, A., Hashemi, S. R., Langroodi, F. R., T, Sadeghi. R., Beyranvand, M.Thrombolytic-plus-Anticoagulant Therapy versus Anticoagulant-Alone Therapy in Submassive Pulmonary Thromboembolism (TVASPE study): a randomized clinical trial. *J. Tehran Heart Cent.* 2014; 9: 104-108.

Teleb, M., Porres-Aguilar, M., Anaya-Ayala, J. E., Rodriguez-Castro, C., Porres-Muñoz, M., Mukherjee, D. Potential role of systemic thrombolysis in acute submassive intermediate risk pulmonary embolism: review and future perspectives. *Ther. Adv. Cardiovasc. Dis.* 2016;10(2):103–10.

Wang, C., Zhai, Z., Yang, Y., Wu, Q., Cheng, Z., Liang, L., Dai, H., Huang, K., Lu, W., Zhang, Z., Cheng, X., Shen, Y.H. Efficacy and safety of low dose recombinant tissue-type plasminogen activator for the treatment of acute pulmonary thromboembolism: a randomized, multicenter, controlled trial. *Chest* 2010; 137:254-62.

Wassef, A., Lim, W., Wu, C. Indications, complications and outcomes of inferior vena cava filters: a retrospective study. *Thromb Res.* 2017; 153: 123-128.

Weitz, J. I., Lensing, A. W A., Prins, M., Bauersachs, R., Beyer-Westendorf, J., Brighton, T.A., Brighton, T. A., Cohen, A. T., Davidson, B. L., Decousus H, Freitas MC, Holberg G. for the EINSTEIN CHOICE Investigators. Rivaroxaban or aspirin for extended treatment of venous thromboembolism. *N Engl. J. Med.* 2017; 376:1211–1222.

Witt, D. M., Nieuwlaat, R., Clark, N. P., Ansell, J., Holbrook, A., Skov, J., Shehab, N., Mock, J., Myers, T., Dentali, F., Crowther, M. A., Agarwal, A., Bhatt, M., Khatib, R., Riva, J. J., Zhang, Y., Guyatt, G. American Society of Hematology 2018 guidelines for management of venous thromboembolism: optimal management of anticoagulation therapy. *Blood Adv.* 2018; 2: 3257-3291.

Chapter 6

Catheter-Directed Treatment of Acute Pulmonary Embolism

Slobodan Obradovic*, PhD
Clinic of Cardiology, Military Medical Academy,
School of Medicine University of Defense, Belgrade, Serbia

Abstract

Acute pulmonary embolism (PE) is a common thromboembolic disease with a wide spectrum of clinical presentation, from asymptomatic to life-threatening shock state with high mortality. Many patients with acute PE have some concomitant disease that can provoke thrombosis or carry a higher bleeding risk. An everyday clinical scenario is patients with high PE mortality risk and high bleeding risk who have contraindications for thrombolytic or anticoagulant therapy. The main purpose of catheter-directed therapy (CDT) in acute PE patients is to diminish the risk of bleeding and to achieve lung reperfusion with either mechanical or chemical means. CDT enables the use of very low doses of thrombolytic therapy with limited bleeding risk, or mechanical fragmentation and aspiration could relieve acute pulmonary trunk obstruction and improve the right ventricle (RV) dysfunction, oxygenation, and hemodynamics. Sometimes it is enough to improve the circulation for only one lobar or a few segmental branches to achieve stabilization. Current guidelines recommend CDT for patients who are at high risk for death from PE due to severe pulmonary artery obstruction with contraindications for systemic thrombolysis or failure of thrombolysis. However, the contemporary approach is closer to using CDT before the overt shock with meticulous, continuous monitoring of the patient's risk. Several

* Corresponding Author's Email: sloba.d.obradovic@gmail.com.

In: Pulmonary Embolism
Editors: Irena Mitevska, Sonja Salinger, Marijan Bosevski et al.
ISBN: 979-8-89113-175-0

devices are available with small trials using soft endpoints of RV status but with encouraging results. The American Heart Association and European Society of Cardiology published their position statements for the use of CDT in acute PE, and the future of this therapy is at the doorstep.

Keywords: acute pulmonary embolism, catheter-directed therapy, thrombolysis, bleeding risk

Introduction

Treatment of acute pulmonary embolism (PE) is often quite challenging. The purpose of catheter-directed therapy (CDT) in acute PE is to reduce obstruction of pulmonary arteries without causing increased bleeding risk. CDT can be used in the form of mechanical fragmentation of thrombus accompanied by thromboaspiration and local application of a lower thrombolytic dose with or without the addition of ultrasound waves in patients with hemodynamic instability. It is expected that both methods will improve the blood flow through pulmonary arteries and improve the patient's outcome. The current guidelines indicated the use of CDT in high-risk PE patients with absolute contraindication to or failed systemic thrombolysis therapy (Konstantinides et al., 2019). This chapter will review the indications and candidates for CDT and the clinical significance of CDT in patients with PE in the light of current clinical data and the Regional Pulmonary Embolism Registry (REPER).

The Need for Catheter-Directed Therapy in Acute Pulmonary Embolism

The majority of patients with acute pulmonary embolism (PE) need only anticoagulant therapy, and they will be cured without any consequences. A relatively small number of patients have severe PE, and the obstruction of the pulmonary tree in them may overcome the adaptive mechanisms and lead to circulatory shock and death (Leidi et al., 2022). The classic therapy for these patients is systemic thrombolytic therapy which is efficient in fast pulmonary reperfusion and can save lives (Leidi et al., 2022; Konstantinides et al., 2019). However, only a small proportion of patients with high-risk PE are treated with systemic thrombolysis (Keller et al., 2020). The main reason for that could be objectively higher risk for bleeding in many of these patients and fear of bleeding in the case of complex patients who are very often old or have several comorbidities (Obradovic et al., 2022). On the other side, some patients with intermediate-high PE risk are at the edge of their capabilities to maintain their hemodynamics, and the outcome of patients with anticoagulant failure is dismal when they undergo hemodynamic breakdown (Furduyna et al., 2018). It is important to recognize the proper moment to prevent circulatory shock and not to wait until it becomes overt. Hence, some patients with intermediate-high-risk PE who do not improve during the first days of anticoagulant therapy and have some delicate signs of deterioration also deserve some kind of reperfusion therapy which can relieve the pulmonary artery obstruction and lead to stabilization of the patient's state (Pruszczyk et al., 2022).

The main goal of catheter-directed therapy (CDT) in acute PE is to diminish pulmonary artery obstruction without increasing the risk of bleeding (Pruszczyk et al., 2022; Giri et al., 2019). There are two main principles of CDT: (1) mechanical fragmentation of thrombus, often with aspiration, and (2) the local application of lower thrombolytic dose with or without ultrasound facilitation. Both of these methods can improve the blood flow through pulmonary arteries and provoke distal thrombus embolization with the downstream obstruction of smaller pulmonary vessels.

The current guidelines (Konstantinides et al., 2019) proposed the use of CDT in patients with high-risk PE who either have an absolute contraindication to systemic thrombolysis or failed to improve on thrombolytic therapy. In patients who are normotensive, guidelines recommend CDT if patients become hemodynamically unstable due to PE. However, the evidence-based data to sustain this recommendation are not available (Pruszczyk et al., 2022; Giri et al., 2019). There are no randomized trials in high-risk PE patients with contraindication to thrombolysis that randomized patients to CDT versus anticoagulant therapy only, or surgical embolectomy. There are also no trials that randomized patients with normotensive PE who become hypotensive to CDT versus surgical embolectomy or rescue thrombolysis.

Some catheter devices are designed for the treatment of acute PE and have relatively small, randomized trials (Table 1) or single-arm trials without the statistical power for hard end-points, which enable authorities to give their permission for further use in acute PE. The devices with trials are presented in Table 1. Position papers about the role of CDT in acute PE were published recently by the American Heart Association (Giri et al., 2019) and European Cardiology Society (Pruzszyk et al., 2022).

Table 1. Devices used for CDT in acute PE and studies

Device and mechanism of action	Trials	Results
Local catheter-directed thrombolytic infusion		
Pig-tail	Case series	
Cragg-McNamara	SUNSET comparison with	No difference in mean
Unifuse	EKOS	reduction of thrombus
Fontain	Case series	score
Local catheter-directed thrombolysis facilitated with ultrasound waves EKOS	ULTIMA, SEATTLE II, OPTALYSE, SUNSET	Reduction in RV/LV ratio with various low doses of tPA
Mechanical with aspiration		
Flow Triever	FLARE	Both single-arm trials,
Indigo	EXTRACT-PE	with reduction of RV/LV ratio
Angiojet	Case series	
Bashir	Case series	
Aspirex	Case series	
AngioVac	Case series	

RV- right ventricle; LV-left ventricle.

SUNSET trial (Avgerinos et al., 2021), ULTIMA trial (Kucher et al., 2014), SEATTLE II trial (Piazza et al., 2015), OPTALYSE trial (Tapson et al., 2019), FLARE trial (Tu et al., 2019), EXTRACT-PE (Sista et al., 2021).

What Kind of Patients Really Need CDT?

The decision for that must be the result of the local pulmonary embolism response team, which should evaluate the risk of dying from PE, risk of bleeding on thrombolysis, and other risks and possibilities according to local expertise. The candidates are patients with acute PE who have high or intermediate-high-risk features at admission, and some factors which preclude safe treatment with full dose thrombolysis or surgical embolectomy, or when surgical treatment is unavailable. It is important to recognize signs of deterioration in patients with intermediate-high-risk PE before hemodynamic collapse becomes developed. Local thrombolysis can achieve sustainable pulmonary reperfusion in a few hours with a dose of tPA less than 25 mg, which has a very weak systemic fibrinolytic effect and thus carries a low risk for bleeding. In the case of high-risk PE, the patient's condition is very unstable, and mechanical devices often cannot extract very large thrombus masses; they can even embolize the opened pulmonary arteries and additionally compromise the patient. It is also important not to forget that all these patients need full anticoagulant therapy for adequate protection against thrombotic extension and early thrombosis recurrence.

One option for the temporary stabilization of patients is to put them on extra-corporal membrane oxygenation (ECMO) therapy and to perform CDT under ECMO (Hobohm et al., 2022).

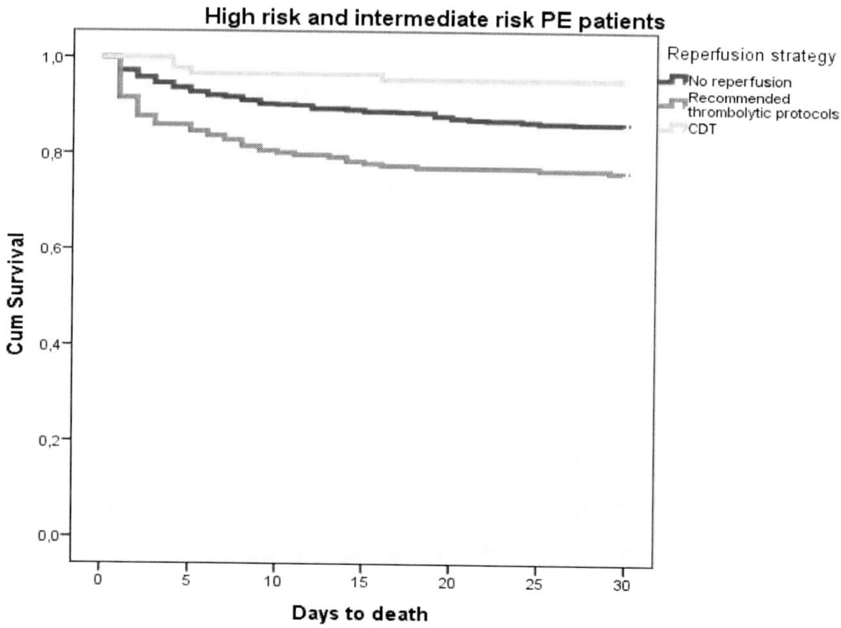

Figure 1. Kaplan-Meier curves of 30-day outcomes of intermediate- and high-risk acute PE patients in respect of the treatment strategy. Results from the regional PE registry on 1016 patients. Log-rank p is less than 0.001.

Results of CDT from the Regional Pulmonary Embolism Registry (REPER)

The regional PE registry is a multicenter, international registry of hospitalized patients enrolled due to acute PE objectively confirmed by computed tomography pulmonary angiography (CTPA). Among 1677 patients enrolled from June 2014–2022, 100 were treated with CDT.

The most often used system was EKOS (53 patients), the pig-tail catheter was used in 45 patients, and the rest used Indigo, Angiojet and Fontain catheters. CDT was used in 90 patients with intermediate- and high-risk PE. CDT was also used in some patients with low-risk PE, in case of pneumonias in the area of occluded pulmonary arteries.

All-cause hospital death was presented with Kaplan-Meiers curves, and a log-rank test was used to determine the difference between therapy modalities. Patients who were treated with slow systemic tPA (it is not a recommended therapy option by the guidelines) protocols and mechanical embolectomy (a small number of patients) were excluded in this analysis.

The maximum dose of tPA given through the catheters was 50 mg, but in the last few years, we adopted the dose according to findings of the OPTALYSE trial, and we used a maximum 25 mg tPA dose with an infusion speed of 1.5–2.5 mg per hour.

The all-cause death from the REPER study in intermediate- and high-risk PE patients was 99/699 (14.2%) in patients who were not treated with reperfusion therapy, 55/227 (24.2%) of patients who received recommended systemic thrombolytic therapy, and 4/90 (4.4%) of patients who underwent CDT (log-rank $p<0.001$) (Figure 1). However, it is clear that patients who received classic thrombolytic therapy represented patients with a higher risk for hospital mortality. The characteristics of patients according to the main therapeutic strategy are presented in Table 1. If we analyzed separately the Kaplan-Meier curves in high-risk PE and intermediate-risk PE the results are as follows: all-cause hospital mortality was 68/613 (11.8%) for no-reperfusion, 22/132 (16.7%) for recommended thrombolytic protocols, and 0/69 (0.0%) for CDT in the intermediate-risk PE subgroup (Log-rank $p=0.002$); and 31/86 (36.0%) for no-reperfusion, 33/95 (34.5%) for recommended thrombolytic protocols, and 4/21 (19.0%) patients treated with CDT in the high-risk PE subgroup (Log-rank $p=0.318$).

Table 2. Characteristics of patients with intermediate- and high-risk PE according to the treatment (results from the regional registry on pulmonary embolism- REPER)

Patient's characteristics	No reperfusion N=699	Recommended thrombolytic protocols N=227	CDT N=90	p
Age – median year (IQR)	69 (60–78)	64 (53–73)	64 (56–73)	<0.001
Female – n, %	384, 54.9	120, 52.9	42 (46.7)	0.319
HR – median beat/min (IQR)	100 (85–115)	110 (97–120)	105 (91–120)	<0.001
SAP – median mmHg (IQR)	120 (105–140)	100 (90–120)	115 (100–130)	<0.001
BNP or NTpBNP – median URL (IQR)	3.3 (1.0–9.5)	3.1 (1.3–7.4)	3.3 (1.6–7.3)	0.969
RVSP – median mmHg (IQR)	45 (36-58)	53 (45–65)	58 (50–70)	<0.001
RVDI – median mm/m^2 median (IQR)	17.5 (15.3–19.8)	20.4 (17.4–22.8)	20.1 (17.7–23.5)	<0.001
GFR – median ml/min (IQR)	65 (43-89)	67 (46–95)	79 (59–100)	<0.001
pO_2 – median mmHg (IQR)	62 (53–76)	61 (49–77)	58 (54–75)	0.388
Intermediate-risk – n, %	613, 87.7	132, 58.1	69, 76.7	<0.001
High-risk – n, %	86, 12.3	95, 41.9	21, 23.3	

HR-heart rate; SAP- systolic arterial pressure; BNP-brain natriuretic peptide; URL-upper reference limit; NTpBNP- N-terminal pro-brain natriuretic peptide; RVSP- right ventricular systolic pressure; RVDI- right ventricular distensibility index; GFR- glomerular filtration rate; IQR-interquartile range; pO_2- partial pressure of oxygen.

There were important differences between the three treatment groups regarding the patients' characteristics, as shown in Table 2. The most important was the proportion of patients in high-risk PE, which is the highest in patients who received recommended thrombolytic protocols with also higher heart rates and lowest arterial systolic pressure at admission in these patients compared to the other two groups. Nevertheless, the aim of this analysis is not a comparison of treatments, but the results of different treatments in certain subgroups of patients. We also can see that the arterial pO_2 and BNP or NT-proBNP increase was not significantly different between groups. Additionally, patients treated with the CDT had the highest right ventricle systolic pressure (RVSP) compared to the other two groups, which indirectly implies the role of cardiac ultrasound in the choice of treatment. The most important result from this study is that no one from the 69 patients in intermediate-high-risk PE treated with CDT died during the hospitalization. The majority of patients in the intermediate-high-risk PE group who were treated with recommended systemic thrombolytic protocols were treated because of the clinical deterioration, and the CDT therapy was used probably earlier in the course of the disease where we can prevent hemodynamic deterioration and have a better outcome. The example of catheter-directed low dose local fibrinolytic therapy in a high-risk young patient with massive PE after spontaneous abortion is shown in Figure 2.

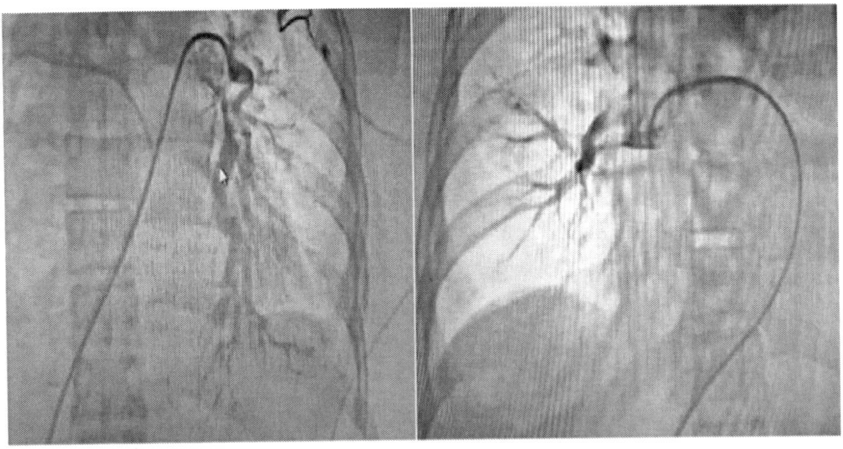

Figure 2. Catheter intervention with local fibrinolytic therapy (tPA 20 mg) in acute massive pulmonary embolism in a high-risk 35 year old patient with Covid-19 infection after spontaneous abortion. Courtesy of Professor Slobodan Obradovic.

Conclusion

CDT is awaiting larger, properly designed studies that will define the place of this approach in the treatment of acute PE patients. Meanwhile, institutions which developed Pulmonary Embolism Response Teams with experience in various treatment modalities will be able to individualize treatment strategies according to risk from PE mortality, risk of bleeding, and risk of other anticipated complications while using different treatments.

Acknowledgments

We acknowledge the significant contribution in the chapter writing by the following physicians: Boris Dzudovic MD, Ph.D., Jovan Matijasevic MD, Ph.D., Uros Batranovic MD, Miodrag Sreckovic MD, Ph.D., Rada Vucic MD, Ph.D., Nebojsa Antonijevic MD, Ph.D.

References

Avgerinos, E. D., Jaber, W., Lacomis, J., Markel, K., McDaniel, M., Rivera-Lebron, B. N., Ross, C. B., Sechrist, J. S., Tom, C., Chaer, R. SUNSET sPE Collaborators. Randomized trial comparing standard versus ultrasound-sssisted thrombolysis for submassive pulmonary embolism: the SUNSET sPE Trial. *JACC Cardiovasc. Interv.* (2021) 14(12):1364-1373.

Furdyna, A., Ciurzynski, M., Roik, M., Paczynska, M., Wretowski, D., Jankowski, K., Lipińska, A., Bienias P, Kosturbiec M, Łabyk A, Trzebicki J, Palczewski P, Kurnicka K, Lichodziejewska B, Pacho S, Pruszczyk P. Management of high risk pulmonary embolism - a single center experience. Folia Med Cracov Folia Med Cracov (2018)58(4):75-83.

Giri, J., Sista, A. K., Weinberg, I., Kearon, C., Kumbhani, D. J., Desai, N. D., Piazza, G., Gladwin, M. T., Chatterjee, S., Kobayashi, T., Kabrhel, C., Barnes, G. D. Interventional therapies for acute Pulmonary embolism: current status and principles for the development of novel evidence: A scientific statement from the American Heart Association. *Circulation* (2019) 140(20):e774-e801.

Hobohm, L., Sagoschen, I., Habertheuer, A, Barco, S., Valerio, L., Wild, J., Schmidt, F. P., Gori, T., Münzel, T., Konstantinides, S., Keller, K. Clinical use and outcome of extracorporeal membrane oxygenation in patients with pulmonary embolism. *Resuscitation* (2022) 170:285-292.

Keller, K., Hobohm, L., Ebner, M., Kresoja, K. P., Münzel T, Konstantinides S. V., Lankeit M. Trends in thrombolytic treatment and outcomes of acute pulmonary embolism in Germany. *Eur. Heart J.* (2020) 41(4):522-529.

Konstantinides, S. V, Meyer, G., Becattini, C., Bueno, H., Geersing, G. J., Harjola, V. P., Huisman, M. V., Humbert, M., Jennings, C. S., Jiménez, D., Kucher, N., Lang, I. M., Lankeit, M., Lorusso, R., Mazzolai, L., Meneveau, N., Áinle, F. N., Prandoni, P., Pruszczyk, P., Righini, M., Torbicki, A., Belle, E. V., Zamorano, J. L.; ESC Scientific Document Group. ESC Guidelines for the diagnosis and management of acute pulmonary embolism developed in collaboration with the European Respiratory Society (ERS). *Eur. Heart J.* 2020 Jan 21;41(4):543-603.

Kucher, N., Boekstegers, P., Muller, O. J., Kupatt, C., Beyer-Westendorf, J., Heitzer, T., Tebbe, U., Horstkotte, J., Müller, R., Blessing, E., Greif, M., Lange, P., Hoffmann, R. T., Werth, S., Barmeyer, A., Härtel, D., Grünwald, H., Empen, K., Baumgartner, I. Randomized, controlled trial of ultrasound-assisted catheter-directed thrombolysis for acute intermediate-risk pulmonary embolism. *Circulation* (2014) 129(4):479-486.

Leidi, A., Bex, S., Righini, M., Berner, A., Grosgurin, O., Marti, C. Risk stratification in patients with acute pulmonary embolism: current evidence and perspectives. *J. Clin. Med.* (2022) 11:2533.

Obradovic, S., Subotic, B., Dzudovic, B., Matijasevic, J., Dzudovic, J., Salinger-Martinovic, S., Miloradovic, V., Kovacevic-Preradovic, T., Marinkovic, J., Neskovic, A.. Pulmonary embolism bleeding score index (PEBSI): A new tool for the detection of patients with low risk for major bleeding on thrombolytic therapy. *Thromb. Res.* (2022) 214:138-143.

Piazza, G., Hohlfelder, B., Jaff, M. R., Ouriel, K., Engelhardt, T. C., Sterling, K. M., Jones, N. J., Gurley, J. C., Bhatheja, R., Kennedy, R. J., Goswami, N., Natarajan, K., Rundback, J., Sadiq, I. R., Liu, S. K., Bhalla, N., Raja, M. L., Weinstock, B. S., Cynamon, J., Elmasri, F. F., Garcia, M. J., Kumar, M., Ayerdi, J., Soukas, P., Kuo, W., Liu, P. Y., Goldhaber, S. Z. SEATTLE II Investigators. A prospective, single-arm, multicenter trial of ultrasound-facilitated, catheter-directed, low-dose fibrinolysis for acute massive and submissive pulmonary embolism: The SEATTLE II study. *JACC Cardiovasc. Interv.* (2015) 8(10):1382-1392.

Pruszczyk, P., Klok, F. A., Kucher, N., Roik, M., Meneveau, N., Sharp, A. S., Nielsen-Kudsk, J. E., Obradović, S., Barco, S., Giannini, F., Stefanini, G., Tarantini, G., Konstantinides, S., Dudek, D. Percutaneous treatment options for acute pulmonary embolism: a position paper of the ESC Working Group on Pulmonary Circulation and Right Ventricular Function and European Association of Percutaneous Cardiovascular Interventions. *Eurointervention* (2022) 18(8):e623-e638.

Sista, A. K., Horowitz, J. M., Tapson, V. F., Rosenberg, M., Elder, M. D., Schiro, B. J., Dohad, S., Amoroso, N. E., Dexter, D. J., Loh, C. T., Leung, D. A., Bieneman, B. K., Perkowski, P. E., Chuang, M. L., Benenati, J. F.; EXTRACT-PE Investigators. Indigo Aspiration System for Treatment of Pulmonary Embolism: Results of the EXTRACT-PE Trial. *JACC Cardiovasc. Interv.* (2021) 14(3):319-329.

Tapson, V. F., Sterling, K., Jones, N., Elder M., Tripathy, U., Brower, J., Maholic, R. M., Ross, C. B., Natarajan, K., Fong, P., Greenspon, L., Tamaddon, H., Piracha, A. R., Engelhardt, T., Katopodis, J., Marques, V., Sharp A. S. P., Piazza, G., Goldhaber, S.

Z. A Randomized Trial of the Optimum Duration of Acoustic Pulse Thrombolysis Procedure in Acute Intermediate-Risk Pulmonary Embolism: The OPTALYSE PE Trial. *JACC Cardiovasc. Interv.* (2018) 11(14):1401-1410.

Tu, T., Toma, C., Tapson V. F., Adams, C., Jaber, W. A., Silver, M., Khandhar S., Amin R., Weinberg, M., Engelhardt, T., Hunter, M., Holmes, D., Hoots, G., Hamdalla H., Maholic, R. L., Lilly, S. M., Ouriel, K., Rosenfield, K.., and for the FLARE Investigators.A prospective, single-arm, multicenter trial of catheter-directed mechanical thrombectomy for intermediate-risk acute pulmonary embolism: the FLARE study. *JACC Cardiovasc. Interv.* (2019) 12(9):859-869.

Chapter 7

Thromboprophylaxis of Venous Thromboembolism

Sonja Salinger[1,*], PhD
and Irena Mitevska[2], PhD
[1]Cardiology Clinic, Clinical Center Nis, Serbia
[2]University Cardiology Clinic, Medical Faculty, Skopje, North Macedonia

Abstract

Venous thromboembolism (VTE) remains highly prevalent in medically ill patients and often leads to increased mortality and cost burden during hospitalization and post-discharge. Nearly half of all VTEs occur during or after hospitalization, with pulmonary embolism accounting for 10% of inpatient mortality. VTE is a common source of perioperative morbidity and mortality and remains a leading direct cause of maternal death in the UK as well. The National Institute for Health and Care Excellence (NICE) estimates that low-molecular-weight heparin (LMWH) reduces VTE risk in medical and surgical patients by 60% and 70%, respectively. Therefore, it is reasonable to assume that it may substantially reduce the risk of VTE in obstetric patients. It has been shown that appropriate prophylaxis in high-risk patients reduces the risk of VTE and related mortality.

Keywords: venous thromboembolism, prophylaxis, acutely ill patients, surgery, obstetrics

---

[*] Corresponding Author's Email: sonja.salinger@gmail.com.

In: Pulmonary Embolism
Editors: Irena Mitevska, Sonja Salinger, Marijan Bosevski et al.
ISBN: 979-8-89113-175-0

Introduction

Venous thromboembolism (VTE) is the third most common cardiovascular diagnosis. Approximately 50% of all VTE events occur as a result of a current or recent hospital admission for surgery or acute medical illness (Schunemann HJ et al., 2018). Hospital-acquired VTE is preventable, with interventions including anticoagulants and mechanical measures, including compression stockings and intermittent pneumatic compression.

Other non-hospitalized medical populations that are at increased risk for VTE include long-term care residents, frail persons, those with minor injuries, and long-distance travelers, particularly those with preexisting VTE risk factors.

Description of the Health Problem

VTE in hospitalized and non-hospitalized medical patients and long-distance travelers confers an important disease burden and can be fatal. Approximately 50% of all VTE events in the community occur as a result of a current or recent hospital admission, mainly for surgery (24%) or acute medical illness (22%). Thus, hospitalization for acute medical illness is an important opportunity for applying prevention efforts. Risk factors for hospital-acquired VTE include acute medical illness, surgery, cancer and cancer therapy, trauma, immobilization, central venous catheters, previous history of VTE, older age, and obesity. Almost all hospitalized patients have one or more risk factors for VTE, and approximately 40% have ≥ 3 risk factors (NICE clinical guideline, 2018). In a United States population-based study, hospital-acquired deep vein thrombosis (DVT) and pulmonary embolism (PE) occurred in 1.3% and 0.4% of hospital admissions, respectively. The increased risk of VTE persists for 45 to 60 days after hospital discharge. Other medical populations that may be at increased risk for VTE include long-term care residents, frail persons, those with minor injuries, and long-distance travelers, particularly those with preexisting VTE risk factors. Medical inpatients are a heterogeneous population in terms of VTE risk, but these patients have conventionally been subject to universal or group-based VTE prevention strategies. Critically ill patients were defined as suffering from an immediately life-threatening condition requiring hospitalization in an intensive or critical care unit. Chronically ill medical patients were defined as those with medical conditions who may be cared for in long-term care facilities. We also considered long-distance travelers, as those traveling by air for > 4 hours and outpatients with minor provoking risk factors for VTE.

Based on an enhanced understanding of these issues, a paradigm shift in VTE risk assessment and prevention is underway that prompts clinicians to strive for individualized prophylaxis based on VTE and bleeding risk. Over prophylaxis of low-risk patients and under prophylaxis of high-risk patients may lead to an unfavorable risk–harm balance for these patients. Over the last decade, several quantitative VTE risk-assessment models (RAMs) were developed for medical inpatients (Stuck et al., 2017). The two most extensively studied are the empirically derived Padua score (Table 1) and the database-derived *International Medical Prevention Registry on Venous Thromboembolism* (IMPROVE) score (Table 2) (Spyropoulos et al., 2011). Both have been externally validated and showed fair discrimination in identifying medical inpatients who are and are not at increased risk for VTE. The IMPROVE investigators also developed an externally validated bleeding risk RAM (Table 3) that may aid in identifying acutely ill medical inpatients at increased risk for bleeding (Decousus et al., 2011). The footnotes of the tables provide data on how these RAMs may be applied for clinical decision-making.

Table 1. Padua VTE RAM score

Padua VTE RAM: score ≥ 4 indicates high VTE risk*	Points
Reduced mobility	3
Active cancer	3
Previous VTE (excluding superficial thrombophlebitis)	3
Known thrombophilic condition	3
Recent trauma or surgery (< 1 month)	2
Elderly age (> 70 years)	1
Heart or respiratory failure	1
Acute myocardial infarction or ischemic stroke	1
Ongoing hormonal treatment	1
Obesity (body mass index > 30)	1
Acute infection or rheumatologic disorder	1

Abbreviations: VTE- venous thromboembolism, RAM- risk-assessment models.

Table 2. IMPROVE VTE RAM score

IMPROVE VTE RAM: score ≥ 2 indicates increased VTE risk†	Points
Previous VTE	3
Known thrombophilia‡	2
Lower limb paralysis§	2
IMPROVE VTE RAM: score ≥ 2 indicates increased VTE risk†	Points
Active cancer	2
Immobilization ≥7d	1
ICU/CCU stay	1
Age >60 years	1

Abbreviations: VTE- venous thromboembolism, ICU/CCU- intensive care unit/coronary care unit.

Table 3. IMPROVE bleeding RAM score

IMPROVE bleeding RAM: score ≥ 7 indicates high bleeding risk	Points
Renal failure (GFR 30–59 vs. ≥ 60 mL/min per m^2)	1
Male vs. female	1
Age 40–80 years vs < 40 years	1.5
Current cancer	2
Rheumatic disease	2
Central venous catheter	2
ICU/Critical Care Unit stay	2.5
Renal failure (GFR < 30 vs. ≥ 60 mL/min per square meter)	2.5
Hepatic failure (INR > 1.5)	2.5
Age ≥85 years vs. <40 years	3.5
Platelet count < 50 3 x 10^9 /L	4
Bleeding in 3 months before admission	4
Active gastroduodenal ulcer	4.5

CI, confidence interval; CCU, Coronary Care Unit; GFR, glomerular filtration rate; ICU, Intensive Care Unit; INR, international normalized ratio. *A total of 60.3% of patients in this study were low-risk (Padua score 0–3). VTE prophylaxis was administered by provider choice from among several medications and with or without concomitant compression stockings.36 VTE incidence without VTE prophylaxis: Padua score 0 to 3: 0.3% Padua score ≥ 4: 11% Among at-risk patients (Padua score ≥ 4) Overall VTE hazard ratio (HR), 32 (95% CI, 4.1–251) Incidence of VTE No prophylaxis: 11% With prophylaxis: 2.2% VTE HR with prophylaxis, 0.13 (95% CI, 0.04–0.4) Incidence of major or clinically relevant nonmajor bleeding with prophylaxis 5 1.6% (95% CI, 0.5–4.6) Interpretation: among at-risk patients (Padua score ≥ 4), the reduction in VTE appears to outweigh the increased risk of bleeding with pharmacologic prophylaxis. †Risk level: score of 0 or 1 5 low risk, score of 2 or 3 5 moderate risk; score ≥ 4 5 high risk. For scores ≥ 2, VTE prophylaxis is indicated. A total of 69% of patients in this study 37 were at low risk for VTE (score 0 or 1). Three-month rate of symptomatic VTE: IMPROVE VTE score 0 or 1: 0.5% IMPROVE VTE score 2 or 3: 1.5% IMPROVE VTE score ≥ 4: 5.7%. ‡Congenital or acquired thrombophilic condition (e.g., factor V Leiden, lupus anticoagulant, protein C, or protein S deficiency). §Leg falls to bed by 5 seconds but has some effort against gravity using the National Institutes of Health stroke scale. {Approximately 90% of patients in this study 40 were low risk for bleeding (score < 7). Incidence of major bleeding/any bleeding: IMPROVE bleeding score < 7: 0.4%/1.5% IMPROVE bleeding score ≥7: 4.1%/7.9%.

Recommendations of VTE prophylaxis in medical inpatients, long-term care residents, persons with minor injuries, and long-distance travelers are summarized in Table 4 (Schunemann et al., 2018).

Table 4. VTE prophylaxis for in/out patients, persons with minor injuries, and long-distance travelers

Acutely ill patients: pharmacological prophylaxis addressing the following comparisons
UFH, LMWH, or fondaparinux rather than no parenteral anticoagulant
LMWH or fondaparinux rather than UFH
These recommendations also apply to anticoagulant choices when VTE prophylaxis is considered for patients with stroke.
Critically ill patients: pharmacological prophylaxis addressing the following comparisons
UFH or LMWH over no UFH or LMWH
In critically ill medical patients, LMWH is preferred over UFH
Acutely or critically ill patients: mechanical prophylaxis addressing the following comparisons
Pharmacological VTE prophylaxis over mechanical VTE prophylaxis.
In acutely or critically ill medical patients who do not receive pharmacological VTE prophylaxis, the mechanical VTE prophylaxis is preferred over no VTE prophylaxis.
Pharmacological or mechanical VTE prophylaxis alone over mechanical combined with pharmacological VTE prophylaxis is suggested.

Table 4. (Continued)

Pneumatic compression devices or graduated compression stockings for VTE prophylaxis in case of mechanical prophylaxis.
DOACs in acutely ill medical patients
LMWH over DOACs as VTE prophylaxis
Inpatient VTE prophylaxis with LMWH only, rather than inpatient and extended duration outpatient VTE prophylaxis with DOACs.
Extended-duration outpatient prophylaxis vs. inpatient-only prophylaxis
In acutely ill medical patient inpatient over inpatient plus extended-duration outpatient VTE prophylaxis is recommended.
In critically ill medical patients, inpatient over inpatient plus extended-duration outpatient VTE prophylaxis is recommended.
Chronically ill patients or nursing home patients
Not using VTE prophylaxis compared with using any VTE prophylaxis is suggested.
Medical outpatients with minor provoking factors for VTE (immobility, minor injury, illness, infection)
VTE prophylaxis is not suggested.
Long-distance travelers: prophylaxis addressing the following comparisons
In long-distance (> 4 hours) travelers without risk factors for VTE, using graduated compression stockings, LMWH, or aspirin for VTE prophylaxis is not suggested.
People without known risk factors who place a high value on prevention of VTE may choose to use graduated compression stockings (also reduce edema).
In substantially increased VTE risk (recent surgery, history of VTE, postpartum women, active malignancy, or ≥ 2 risk factors, including combinations of the above with hormone replacement therapy, obesity, or pregnancy), graduated compression stockings or prophylactic LMWH are suggested.
In substantially increased VTE risk (recent surgery, history of VTE, postpartum women, active malignancy, or ≥ 2 risk factors, including combinations of the above with hormone replacement therapy, obesity, or pregnancy) and in whom LMWH or graduated compression stockings are not feasible (resource-constrained setting or aversion to other indicated anticoagulants), aspirin is suggested over no VTE prophylaxis.

Abbreviations: LMWH-low molecular weight heparin; UFH-unfractionated heparin; DOACs- direct oral anticoagulants; VTE-venous thromboembolism.

Prevention of Venous Thromboembolism in Surgical Hospitalized Patients

Deep vein thrombosis (DVT) and pulmonary embolism (PE) (collectively, VTE) are well-recognized, clinically important, and potentially devastating complications that may occur following major surgical procedures, defined as any surgical intervention that carries greater than minimal risk, is performed in the operating room, and requires specialized training. Before the era of the routine use of effective prophylaxis, VTE was a common cause of morbidity and mortality following major surgery. It has been estimated to cause > 50,000 deaths per annum in the United States alone. The importance of preventative measures to minimize the risk of VTE following major surgery has been recognized for decades; however, even with the use of prophylaxis, surgery accounts for approximately 25% of VTEs observed in communities (Anderson et al., 2019). Although most surgical procedures carry some risk for VTE, this risk varies considerably across surgical procures and among individual patients undergoing surgery. Surgical procedures carrying the highest risk of developing postoperative VTE include hip and knee arthroplasty, invasive neurosurgical procures, and major vascular procedures. Patient factors that carry greater risks for thrombosis include histories of VTE, particularly if unprovoked or associated with cancer, or cancer, even in the absence of previous VTE. Scoring systems that calculate the risk of postoperative VTE for individual patients, such as the Caprini score, have been developed and validated following some surgical procedures (Caprini et al., 2005). Although postoperative VTE has historically been a complication primarily occurring in the hospital, with shortened hospital stays, postoperative VTE often occurs in the days to weeks following discharge from the hospital.

Recommendations of VTE prophylaxis in patients hospitalized for major surgical interventions, including orthopedic, major neurosurgery, urological, vascular, trauma, gynecology, and general major surgeries are summarized in the following tables (Tables 5–11).

Table 5. VTE prophylaxis in patients hospitalized for major surgical intervention

Perioperative VTE prophylaxis in major surgery in general
Pharmacological or mechanical prophylaxis is suggested
In high bleeding risk, mechanical methods may be favorable over pharmacological prophylaxis.
In patients who do not receive pharmacologic prophylaxis, mechanical prophylaxis over no mechanical prophylaxis is suggested.
In the case of mechanical prophylaxis, intermittent compression devices over graduated compression stockings are suggested.
In patients on pharmacologic prophylaxis, combined prophylaxis with mechanical and pharmacological methods over prophylaxis with pharmacological agents alone is suggested.
In the case of high risk for VTE, combined prophylaxis is favored over mechanical or pharmacological prophylaxis alone.
Combined mechanical and pharmacological prophylaxis or mechanical prophylaxis alone, depending on the risk of VTE and bleeding based on the individual patient and the type of surgical procedure, is suggested.
For patients considered at high risk for VTE, combined prophylaxis is particularly favored over mechanical or pharmacological prophylaxis alone.
For patients undergoing major surgery, the American Society of Hematology guideline panel suggests against using IVC filters for prophylaxis of VTE.
Extended antithrombotic prophylaxis over short-term antithrombotic prophylaxis is suggested.
Extended prophylaxis was generally considered as beyond 3 weeks (range: 19–42 days), and short-term prophylaxis was considered as up to 2 weeks (range: 4–14 days).
Early or delayed antithrombotic prophylaxis is suggested.

Abbreviations: VTE-venous thromboembolism; IVC- inferior vena cava.

Table 6. VTE prophylaxis in patients hospitalized for orthopedic surgery

For total hip arthroplasty or total knee arthroplasty, ASA or anticoagulants are suggested.
For total hip arthroplasty or total knee arthroplasty DOACs over LMWH are suggested.
Any of the DOACs approved for use are suggested.
If a DOAC is not used, LMWH is suggested rather than warfarin.

If a DOAC is not used, LMWH is suggested rather than UFH.
For hip fracture repair, pharmacological prophylaxis over no pharmacological prophylaxis is suggested.
For hip fracture repair, LMWH or UFH are suggested.

Abbreviations: LMWH-low molecular weight heparin; UFH-unfractionated heparin; DOACs- direct oral anticoagulants; ASA- acetylsalicylic acid.

Table 7. VTE prophylaxis in patients hospitalized for major general surgery

Pharmacological prophylaxis over no pharmacological prophylaxis is suggested.
LMWH or UFH are suggested.
For laparoscopic cholecystectomy, pharmacological prophylaxis is not suggested.
In case of other risk factors for VTEs (e.g., history of VTE, thrombophilia, or malignancy) pharmacological prophylaxis may be beneficial.

Abbreviations: LMWH-low molecular weight heparin; UFH-unfractionated heparin; VTE-venous thromboembolism.

Table 8. VTE prophylaxis in patients hospitalized for major neurosurgical procedures

Pharmacological prophylaxis is not suggested.
Prophylaxis with mechanical methods is suggested.
Pharmacological prophylaxis may be warranted in a higher-risk subgroup of patients with prolonged immobility following surgery.
Pharmacological prophylaxis could be considered for patients undergoing major neurosurgical procedures that carries a lower risk for major bleeding and in those patients with persistent mobility restrictions after the bleeding risk declines following surgery.
In patients on pharmacological prophylaxis, LMWH over UFH is suggested.

Abbreviations: LMWH - low molecular weight heparin; UFH - unfractionated heparin.

Table 9. VTE prophylaxis in patients hospitalized for urological procedures

For TURP, pharmacological prophylaxis is not suggested.
Patients with other risk factors for VTE (e.g., history of VTE, thrombophilia, or malignancy) may benefit from pharmacological prophylaxis.

Table 9. (Continued)

For TURP, when pharmacological prophylaxis is used, LMWH or UFH are suggested.
For radical prostatectomy, pharmacological prophylaxis is not suggested.
For extended node dissection or open radical prostatectomy. pharmacological prophylaxis may be potentially beneficial.
For radical prostatectomy and use of pharmacological prophylaxis, LMWH or UFH are suggested.

Abbreviations: LMWH-low molecular weight heparin; UFH-unfractionated heparin; VTE-venous thromboembolism; TURP - transurethral resection of the prostate.

Table 10. VTE prophylaxis in patients with cardiac or major vascular surgery

Pharmacological prophylaxis or no pharmacological prophylaxis are suggested.
When pharmacological prophylaxis is used, LMWH or UFH are suggested.

Abbreviations: LMWH-low molecular weight heparin; UFH-unfractionated heparin.

Table 11. VTE prophylaxis in patients hospitalized for major trauma

In low to moderate bleeding risk, pharmacological prophylaxis is suggested.
In high bleeding risk, pharmacological prophylaxis is not suggested.
For patients experiencing major trauma in whom pharmacological prophylaxis is used, LMWH or UFH are suggested.

Abbreviations: LMWH-low molecular weight heparin; UFH-unfractionated heparin.

Table 12. VTE prophylaxis in patients hospitalized for major gynecological surgery

Pharmacological prophylaxis over no pharmacological prophylaxis is suggested.
LMWH or UFH are suggested.

Abbreviations: LMWH-low molecular weight heparin; UFH-unfractionated heparin.

Obstetric Thromboprophylaxis Risk Assessment and Management

Antenatal Assessment and Management

All women should undergo a documented assessment of risk factors for VTE in early pregnancy or pre-pregnancy. Risk assessment should be repeated if the woman is admitted to the hospital for any reason or develops other intercurrent problems. Risk assessment should be repeated intrapartum or immediately postpartum. Any woman with four or more current risk factors shown in Table 13 (other than previous VTE or thrombophilia) should be considered for prophylactic LMWH throughout the antenatal period and will usually require prophylactic LMWH for 6 weeks postnatally, but a postnatal risk reassessment should be made. Any woman with three current risk factors shown in Table 6 (other than previous VTE or thrombophilia) should be considered for prophylactic LMWH from 28 weeks and will usually require prophylactic LMWH for 6 weeks postnatally, but a postnatal risk reassessment should be made. Any woman with two current risk factors shown in Table 6 (other than previous VTE or thrombophilia) should be considered for prophylactic LMWH for at least 10 days postpartum. Women admitted to the hospital when pregnant (including to the gynecology ward with hyperemesis gravidarum or ovarian hyperstimulation syndrome) should usually be offered thromboprophylaxis with LMWH unless there is a specific contraindication such as the risk of labor or active bleeding (Tables 12–14). The risk of VTE should be discussed with women at risk, and the reasons for individual recommendations explained (RCOG, 2015).

Table 13. Antenatal assessment and management (to be assessed at booking and repeated if admitted)

Any previous VTE except a single event related to major surgery	HIGH RISK – requires antenatal prophylaxis with LMWH
Hospital admission	INTERMEDIATE RISK Consider antenatal prophylaxis with LMWH
Single previous VTE related to major surgery	
High-risk thrombophilia + no VTE	

Table 13. (Continued)

Any previous VTE except a single event related to major surgery	HIGH RISK – requires antenatal prophylaxis with LMWH
Medical comorbidities (cancer, heart failure, active SLE, IBD or inflammatory polyarthropathy, nephrotic syndrome, type I DM with nephropathy, sickle cell disease, current IVDU	
Any surgical procedure e.g., appendicectomy	
OHSS (first trimester only)	
Obesity (BMI >30 kg/m^2)	Four or more risk factors: prophylaxis from first trimester
Age > 35	
Parity ≥3	
Smoker	
Gross varicose veins	
Current pre-eclampsia	Three risk factors: prophylaxis from 28 weeks
Immobility, e.g., paraplegia, PGP	
Family history of unprovoked or estrogen-provoked VTE in a first-degree relative	
Low-risk thrombophilia	LOWER RISK Fewer than three risk factors: Mobilization and avoidance of dehydration
Multiple pregnancies	
IVF/ART	
Transients risk factors: Dehydration/hyperemesis; current systemic infection; long-distance travel	

Abbreviations: APL-antiphospholipid antibodies (lupus anticoagulants, anticardiolipin antibodies, P2-glycoprotein 1 antibodies); ART-assisted reproductive technology; BMI based on booking weight; DM-diabetes mellitus; FHx - family history; gross varicose veins-symptomatic, above knee or associated with phlebitis/edema/skin changes; high-risk thrombophilia-antithrombin deficiency, protein C or S deficiency, compound or homozygous for low-risk thrombophilia's; IBD-inflammatory bowel disease; immobility- ≥ 3 days; IVDU-intravenous drug user; IVF-in vitro fertilization; LMWH-low molecular weight heparin; long-distance travel-> 4 hours; low-risk thrombophilia-heterozygous for factor V Leiden or prothrombin G20210A mutations; OHSS-ovarian hyperstimulation syndrome; PGP-pelvic girdle pain with reduced mobility; PPH-postpartum hemorrhage; thrombophilia-inherited or acquired; VTE-venous thromboembolism; SLE- systemic lupus erythematosus; BMI- body mass index.

Table 14. Postnatal assessment and management (to be assessed in the delivery suite)

Any previous VTE Anyone requiring antenatal LMWH Hospital admission High-risk thrombophilia Low-risk thrombophilia + FHx	HIGH RISK At least 6 weeks postnatal prophylactic LMWH
Cesarean section in labor BMI ≥40 kg/m² Readmission or prolonged admission (≥3 days) in the puerperium Any surgical procedure in the puerperium except immediate repair of the perineum Medical comorbidities e.g., cancer, heart failure, active SLE, IBD or inflammatory polyarthropathy, nephrotic syndrome, type I DM with nephropathy, sickle cell disease, current IVDU	INTERMEDIATE RISK At least 10 days postnatal prophylactic LMWH NB if persisting or >3 risk factors consider extending thromboprophylaxis with LMWH
Age > 35 years Obesity (BMI >30 kg/m²) Parity ≥3 Smoker Elective cesarean section Family history of VTE Low-risk thrombophilia Gross varicose veins Current systemic infection Immobility (paraplegia, PGP, long-distance travel) Current pre-eclampsia Multiple pregnancy Preterm delivery in this pregnancy (<37th weeks) Stillbirth in this pregnancy Mid-cavity rotational or operative delivery Prolonged labor (> 24 hours) PPH > 1 liter or blood transfusion	Two or more risk factors: INTERMEDIATE RISK Fewer than two risk factors: LOWER RISK Early mobilization and avoidance of dehydration

Abbreviations: BMI- body mass index; DM-diabetes mellitus; FHx - family history; gross varicose veins-symptomatic, above knee or associated with phlebitis/edema/skin changes; high-risk thrombophilia-antithrombin deficiency, protein C or S deficiency, compound or homozygous for low-risk thrombophilia's; IBD-inflammatory bowel disease; immobility- ≥ 3 days; IVDU-intravenous drug user; IVF-in vitro fertilization; LMWH-low molecular weight heparin; VTE-venous thromboembolism; SLE- systemic lupus erythematosus.

Antenatal and postnatal prophylactic dose of LMWH:

Weight< 50 kg = 20 mg enoxaparin/2500 units dalteparin/3500 units tinzaparin daily
Weight 50–90 kg = 40 mg enoxaparin/5000 units dalteparin/4500 units tinzaparin daily
Weight 91–130 kg = 60 mg enoxaparin/7500 units dalteparin/7000 units tinzaparin daily
Weight 131–170 kg = 80 mg enoxaparin/10000 units dalteparin/9000 units tinzaparin daily
Weight > 170 kg = 0.6 mg/kg/day enoxaparin/75 u/kg/day dalteparin/75 u/kg/days tinzaparin daily

Conclusion

Pharmacological VTE prophylaxis is strongly recommended in acutely or critically ill inpatients at acceptable bleeding risk. If a bleeding risk is unacceptable mechanical prophylaxis is indicated. Direct oral anticoagulants are not recommended during hospitalization as well as extending pharmacological prophylaxis after hospital discharge. In outpatients with minor VTE risk factors, conditional recommendations included not to use VTE prophylaxis routinely in long-term care patients. For long-distance travelers, if they are at high risk for VTE, graduated compression stockings or low molecular weight heparin are conditionally recommended.

References

Anderson, D. R., Morgano, G. P., Bennett, C., Dentali, F., Francis, C. W., Garcia, D. A., Kahn, S.R., Rahman, M., Rajasekhar, A., Rogers, F. B., Smythe, M.A. S., Tikkinen, K. A. O., Yates, A. J., Baldeh, T., Balduzzi, S., Brożek, J. L., Etxeandia-Ikobaltzeta, I., Johal, H., Neumann, I., Wiercioch, W., Yepes-Nuñez, J. J., Schünemann, H. J., Dahm. P. American Society of Hematology 2019 guidelines for management of venous thromboembolism: prevention of venous thromboembolism in surgical hospitalized patients. *Blood Adv* (2019) 3 (23): 3898–3944.

Caprini, J. A. Thrombosis risk assessment as a guide to quality patient care. *Dis. Mon.* 2005;51(2-3):70-78.

Decousus, H., Tapson, V. F., Bergmann, J. F., Chong, B. H., Froehlich, J. B., Kakkar, A. K., Merli, G. J., Monreal, M., Nakamura, M., Pavanello, R., Pini, M., Piovella, F., Spencer, F.A., Spyropoulos, A.C., Turpie, A. G. G., Zotz, R. B., Fitzgerald, G., Anderson, F. A.; IMPROVE Investigators. Factors at admission associated with bleeding risk in medical patients: findings from the IMPROVE investigators. *Chest.* 2011;139(1):69-79.

National Institute for Health and Clinical Excellence. NICE clinical guideline 92: Venous thromboembolism: reducing the risk. http://www.1000livesplus. wales.nhs.uk/ sitesplus/documents/1011/CG92NICEGuidelinePDF.pdf. Accessed 15 April 2018.

Royal College of Obstetricians and Gynaecologist. Reducing the Risk of Venous Thromboembolism during Pregnancy and the Puerperium. *Green-top Guideline* No. 37a April 2015.

Schunemann, H. J., Cushman, M., Burnett, A. E., Kahn, S. R., Beyer-Westendorf, J., Spencer, F. A., Rezende, S. M., Zakai, N. A., Bauer, K, A., Dentali, F., Lansing, J., Balduzzi, S., Darzi, A., Morgano, G. P., Neumann, I., Nieuwlaat, R., Yepes-Nuñez, J. J., Zhang, Y., Wiercioch, W. American Society of Hematology 2018 guidelines for management of venous thromboembolism: prophylaxis for hospitalized and nonhospitalized medical patients. *Blood Adv.* (2018) 2 (22): 3198–3225.

Spyropoulos, A. C., Anderson, F. A., FitzGerald, G., Decousus, H., Pini, M., Chong, B. H., Zotz, R. B., Bergmann, J. F., Tapson, V., Froehlich, J. B., Monreal, M., Merli, G. J., Pavanello, R., Turpie, A. G. G., Nakamura, M., Piovella, F., Kakkar, A. K., Spencer, F.A.; IMPROVE Investigators; IMPROVE Investigators. Predictive and associative models to identify hospitalized medical patients at risk for VTE. *Chest.* 2011;140(3):706-714.

Stuck, A. K., Spirk, D., Schaudt, J., Kucher, N. Risk assessment models for venous thromboembolism in acutely ill medical patients. A systematic review. *Thromb Haemost.* 2017 Apr 3;117(4):801-808.

Chapter 8

Deep Venous Thrombosis: Diagnosis and Treatment

Marijan Bosevski[*]**, PhD**
University Cardiology Clinic, St. Cyril and Methodius University,
Faculty of Medicine, Skopje, North Macedonia

Abstract

Deep venous thrombosis is a clinical entity that accompanies the pathological substrate of thrombi in the venous systemic circulation. After assessment of the probability for its occurrence upon presence of symptoms, signs, and risk factors, diagnosis is made by ultrasound. Therapeutic modalities with standard and novel direct anticoagulants (DOACs) are discussed in this chapter.

Keywords: deep venous thrombosis, diagnosis, anticoagulation

Introduction

The frequency of deep venous thrombosis (DVT), according to Cohen, is calculated as incidence of 148 per 1000 inhabitants, i.e., for pulmonary thromboembolism. The incidence increases with age and the number of comorbidities. Several factors participate in the formation of the thrombus (Table 1). All of them enter at least one of the links of the pathological triad of Virchow: hypercoagulability, vascular injury, or venous stasis. Despite the

[*] Corresponding Author's Email: marijanbosevski@yahoo.com.

In: Pulmonary Embolism
Editors: Irena Mitevska, Sonja Salinger, Marijan Bosevski et al.
ISBN: 979-8-89113-175-0

epidemiological knowledge about venous thromboembolism (VTE), almost one-third of these patients have no recognized risk factor. Twenty percent of all cases of VTE are due to malignant diseases, and 15% to a large surgery or prolonged immobilization. The "medical" patients or those with heart failure, respiratory failure, or myocardial infarction with complications are high-risk patients, despite the previous one's classifications, because their prognosis depends on the occurrence of DVT or PE, which develops as a complication (Wendelboe et al., 2016).

The importance of risk factors is assessed based on probability, the same to cause VTE. Accordingly, in Table 1 are given the predisposing factors for VTE, classified according to their significance.

Table 1. Wells score, applicable to DVT

Factors	Points
Active Cancer	+1
Bedridden recent, ≥3 days, or major surgery within 12 weeks	+1
Swelling > 3 cm relative to the other leg	+1
Collateral superficial veins	+1
Swelling of whole leg	+1
Localized changes along a deep vein	+1
Edema of the opposite leg, limited to the symptomatic leg	+1
Paralysis or recent immobilization of the lower extremity	+1
Previously documented deep vein thrombosis	+1
An alternative diagnosis of DVT, which is more likely than the first	-2

Low probability < 1, moderate 1–2, likely > 2, high probability ≥ 3.
Adapted from Bosevski et al., Vein thrombology.

The score is not applicable to hospitalized patients.

The D-dimer test is used as a test to rule out VTE. The universal cut point for D-dimer values does not exist because it depends on the test used for D-dimer evaluation. A value above 500 ng/mL has diagnostic significance. In patients over 50, the cut-off is calculated as years multiplied by ten. The Elisa D-dimer test or immunoturbidimetric test are the preferred tests for diagnosis of DVT.

Clinical Symptoms and Signs

Swelling of the limb is often present in the distal part or all over the limb while its contours have been changed. The extremity is red, painful, and warm. Peripheral swelling occurs acutely and is unilateral, not testicular, which makes a difference regarding cardiac edema and hypoalbuminemia. The differential diagnosis is also made in relation to the superficial thrombophlebitis, where there is localized redness and swelling, and the superficial one's veins are palpated as hard red-livid bundles, i.e., post-thrombotic syndrome, where the skin is atrophic, cold with defects and ulcerations.

Clinical-Diagnostic Approach

The diagnosis of deep vein thrombosis is based on vascular ultrasound imaging. Venous ultrasound is a method as the first line imaging modality in the diagnosis of DVT (Goodacre et al., 2005). Ultrasound (Echo color Doppler sonography) reveals incompressibility of the affected vein, loss of respiratory phase signal, but also the absence of signal and visualization of the thrombus in various stages, as a direct sign (Figures 1 and 2).

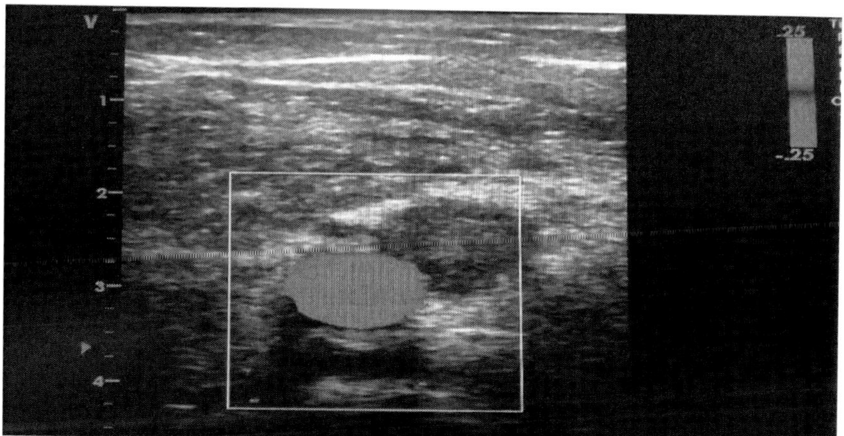

Bosevski M et al., 2016.

Figure 1. Occlusive thrombus in the popliteal vein.

Repeated ultrasound examinations increase the positive predictive value of this method in the detection of DVT. This method has high sensitivity and specificity (over 90%), unlike the D-dimer test which has, above all, a high negative predictive value in relation to the diagnosis of VTE. Considering that 70% of patients with symptomatic PE have DVT, and patients with scan-documented DVT have a 30-70% probability for PE, then pictorial proof of the existence of either form is needed in VTE patients with the given symptoms from one entity. Both imaging methods also have prognostic significance, whether the clinical manifestation is systemically embolized DVT, or whether a PE has visible evidence of its occurrence, i.e., DVT (Figures 1 and 2). A diagnostic algorithm for DVT is shown in Figure 3, adapted from the European Society of Cardiology 2022 consensus on deep vein thrombosis. The therapeutic approach to deep vein thrombosis is identical to that of VTE (Mazzolai et al., 2022). The anticoagulation approach and treatment duration is shown in Figure 4. Monitoring the treatment of DVT has clinical significance considering the outcomes in patients with PE, although the presence of DVT in patients with VTE has no prognostic significance for these patients.

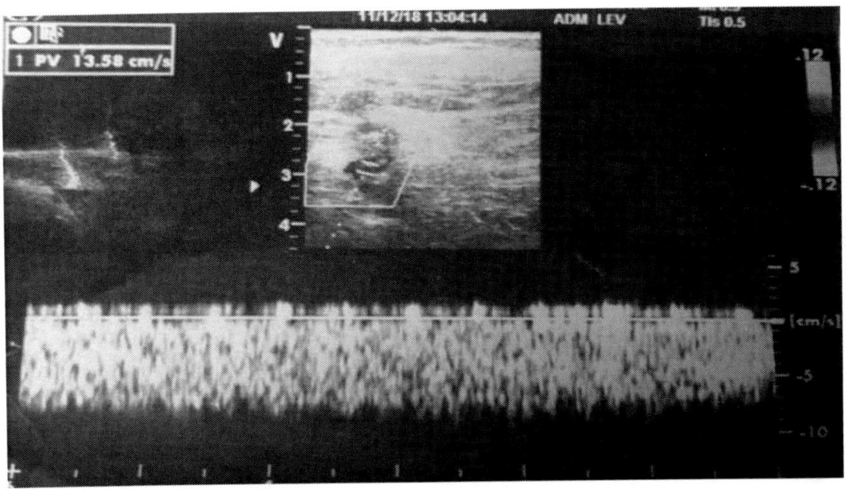

Bosevski M et al., 2016.

Figure 2. Continuous signal as an indirect sign of thrombosis.

Compression stockings have a symptomatic effect in patients with DVT from the time the swelling starts to go down, although randomized Kahn's study has no influence on the occurrence of post-thrombotic syndrome.

Conditions that are an absolute or relative indication for hospitalization treatment of VTE (according to Wells and Spiropolus) are - advanced age, impaired mental status, comorbidities including heart failure and renal and respiratory failure, active or recent bleeding, hemodynamic instability, drug intolerance, thrombophilia, thrombocytopenia (including heparin-induced), massive BE and high (iliofemoral) DVT, need for fibrinolysis, uncontrolled arterial hypertension, recent bleeding or surgery, obesity or low body weight (with the need for an adequate dose of medicine). There are three stages of anticoagulation by Kearon C et al., 2012.

Acute treatment = first 5–7 days, Long-term = 3–6 m, Extended = 6–18 m.

For anticoagulation in non-cancer patients, as already reported in the 2017 edition of ESC consensus on DVT, DOACs should be preferred as first-line anticoagulant therapy in the absence of contraindication.1 However, for patients with COVID-19 infection, particularly in hospitalized patients DOACs should be avoided and parenteral anticoagulation, with unfractionated heparin (UFH) or low-molecular-weight heparin (LMWH), is preferred because of potential high risk of rapid clinical deterioration with multi-organ failure. In addition, concomitant therapy with antiviral agents, immunomodulatory agents, or other investigational treatment have potential drug–drug interactions. Patients with distal (infrapopliteal) DVT treated with anticoagulation vs. placebo showed similar outcomes according to the *anticoagulant* therapy for the symptomatic calf deep vein thrombosis (CACTUS) trial. Only high-risk patients with distal DVT (unprovoked one, with previous history of VTE, carcinoma-associated DVT, advanced age, coexistent medical disease) should be anticoagulated.

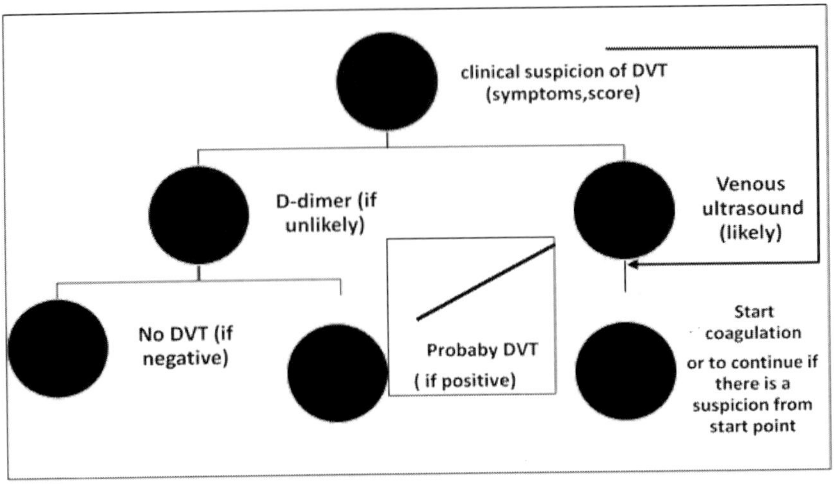

Adapted from European Society of Cardiology Consensus on deep vein thrombosis 2022.

Figure 3. Diagnostic algorithm for deep vein thrombosis.

Catheter-directed in situ thrombolysis (CDT) plus anticoagulation is an effective treatment for proximal DVT but should be reserved for severe cases (CAVA trial).

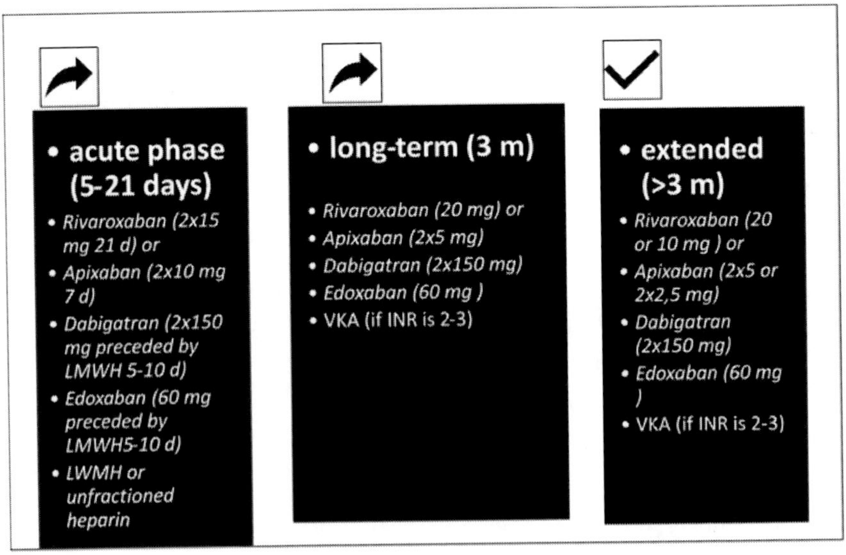

Figure 4. Anticoagulation algorithm.

When anticoagulation is contraindicated in a patient with proximal DVT or in the case of a recurrent episode of DVT/VTE event under adequate therapeutic anticoagulation, vena cava filtering should be considered. To control symptoms of DVT, bandages or compression should also be considered in the first 24 hours (Avila et al., 2019).

Extended anticoagulation means therapy beyond 3 months. It is an individual decision of the physician after assessment of the patient's risk of recurrence, bleeding, and compliance with the drug. Many risk scores, such as VIENNA, HERDOOD2, or DAMOVES, incorporate D-dimer value, male sex, age, localization of thrombi (1st one), clinical signs of DVT (2nd one), and thrombophilia (3rd). In general, high-risk patients with 2 or more risk factors and low risk for bleeding are appropriate candidates for extended treatment (Mai et al., 2019).

Superficial Thrombophlebitis

Superficial thrombophlebitis (SVT) is one of the most common diseases in venous pathology, which is manifested by the presence of a thrombus in the lumen of a superficial vein, which is followed by inflammatory changes in the vein wall and adjacent tissue structures. It is clinically manifested by the presence of a painful, thickened, hardened vein and reddened skin over it. Systemic inflammatory signs can often be present. It most often affects the superficial veins of the lower extremities, but any superficial veins of the body can be affected. SVT is a relatively common disease, but the exact incidence and prevalence of the disease are not known and are likely to be underestimated. Slowed and turbulent blood flow in dilated, morphologically altered superficial veins is most likely the main risk factor within Virchow's triad, which contributes to the occurrence of PT. The retrograde flow of venous blood in the varicose veins, which is a consequence of the disturbed function of the venous valves, as well as the turbulent blood flow, cause immediate damage to the wall of the venous blood vessel, primarily to the venous endothelium, which is responsible for the initiation of the thrombotic process. Superficial thrombophlebitis, which occurs in functionally and morphologically normal veins without varicose changes, is a heterogeneous group of conditions in which the inflammatory and thrombotic processes are expressed differently. This group of diseases includes various autoimmune and systemic diseases of the connective tissue, such as Burger's disease, Bechet's disease, systemic lupus erythematosus (SLE), and other rheumatological diseases, as well as various vasculitis (polyarteritis nodosa, Takayasu arteritis, and Mondor's disease). The background of PT can be a variety of hematological diseases such as essential thrombocytosis, primary or secondary polycythemia, leukemias, lymphomas, and cryoglobulinemia. Furthermore, the ultrasound examination allows us to estimate the distance of the blood thrombus from the saphenous-femoral or saphenous-popliteal mouth, which is of particular importance for determining the risk of spreading the thrombus in the deep system and thus for the selection of optimal therapy, as well as for ruling out the possible presence of simultaneous deep venous thrombosis.

Ultrasound diagnosis is actually based on the same principles that are used in the diagnosis of DVT. LMWH and fondaparinux are reserved for treatment of SVT. In the latest guidelines for the prevention of venous thromboembolisms, the American Society of Thoracic Surgeons recommends treatment of symptomatic SVT (at least 5 cm in length) with fondaparinux or low molecular weight heparin in a preventive dose for a duration of at least 4 weeks, but the recommendation is still based on a low degree of evidence. 3,4 Superficial thrombophlebitis, in which the proximal end of the thrombus approaches less than 3 cm from the saphenous/femoral orifice, is treated in accordance with the guidelines for the treatment of deep vein thrombosis (Kalodiki et al., 2012).

Cancer-Associated Thrombosis (CAT)

Low-molecular-weight heparin is superior to unfractionated heparin in acute phase treatment and superior to VKA in intermediate and prolonged management of PE in CAT. NOAC (Edoxaban, Rivaroxaban, and Apixaban) have equivalent efficacy to LMWH in CAT (Hokusai, Select-D, Carravagio). A detailed treatment approach in CAT is described in Chapter 10.

Conclusion

Deep venous thrombosis is a serious condition that needs prompt diagnosis and decision for early coagulation. The prognosis of patients with DVT complicated by pulmonary thromboembolism is worse compared to patients with isolated DVT. Long-term prognosis of these patients depends on etiology, time of diagnosis, and occurrence of post-thrombotic syndrome.

References

Avila, M. L., Montoya, M., Lumia, C., Marson, A., Brandao, L. R., Tomlinson, G. Compression stockings to prevent post-thrombotic syndrome in adults, a Bayesian meta-analysis. *Thromb. Res.* 2019;182:20–26.

Bosevski, M., Poredos, P., Velkova, E., Spirkoska, A., Kozareva, K. G., Stojanovski, Z. Venous thrombology. *Ars Lamina*, Skopje 2016.

Goodacre, S., Sampson, F., Thomas, S., van Beek, E., Sutton, A. Systematic review and meta-analysis of the diagnostic accuracy of ultrasonography for deep vein thrombosis. *BMC Med. Imaging* 2005; 3:6.

Kalodiki, E., Svrtinova, V., Allegra, C., Andreozii, G., Antignani, P. L., Avram, R., Brkljacic, B., Cadariou, F., Dzsinich, C., Fareed, J., Gaspar, L., Geroulakos, G., Jawien, A., Kozak, M., Lattimer, C. R., Minar, E., Partsch, H., Passariello, F., Patel, M., Pécsvárady, Z., Poredos, P., Roztocil, K., Scuderi, A., Sparovec, M., Szostek,. M, Skorski, M. Superficial vein thrombosis; a consensus statement. *Int. Angiol.* 2012; 31(30:203-16.

Kearon, C., Akl, E. A., Comerota, A. J., Prandoni, P., Bounameaux, H., Goldhaber, S. Z., Nelson, M. E., Wells, P. S., Gould, M. K., Dentali, F., Crowther, M., Kahn, S. R. Antithrombotic therapy for VTE disease: Antithrombotic Therapy and Prevention of Thrombosis, 9th ed: American College of Chest Physicians Evidence-Based Clinical Practice Guidelines. *Chest*, 2012 Feb;141(2 Suppl):e419S-e496S.

Mai, V., Bertoletti, L., Cucherat, M., Jardel, S., Grange, C., Provencher, S., Lega, J. C. Extended anticoagulation for the secondary prevention of venous thromboembolic events: An updated network meta-analysis. *PLoS One* 2019;14: e0214134.

Mazzolai, L., Ageno, W., Alatri, A., Bauersachs, R., Becattini, C., Brodmann, M., Emmerich, J., Konstantinides, S., Meyer, G., Middeldorp. S., Monreal, M., Righini, M., Aboyans, V. Second consensus document on diagnosis and management of acute deep vein thrombosis: updated document elaborated by the ESC Working Group on aorta and peripheral vascular diseases and the ESC Working Group on pulmonary circulation and right ventricular function. *Eur. J. Prev. Cardiol.* 2022 May 27;29(8):1248-1263.

Wendelboe, A. M, Raskob, G. E. Global Burden of Thrombosis: Epidemiologic Aspects. *Circ. Res.* 2016;118(9):1340-7.

Chapter 9

Chronic Thromboembolic Pulmonary Hypertension (CTEHP): Diagnosis, Follow-Up, and Prognosis

Elizabeta Srbinovska Kostovska*, **PhD**
University Clinic of Cardiology, Medical faculty, Skopje, North Macedonia

Abstract

Chronic thromboembolic pulmonary hypertension (CTEPH) is a rare but progressive and potentially life-threatening disease that mainly occurs as an uncommon sequel of acute pulmonary embolism (PE), with a cumulative incidence of 0.9–9.1% within 2 years after an acute PE. Predisposing factors, such as infection, chronic inflammatory diseases, hypothyroidism, malignancy, the presence of antiphospholipid antibodies, elevated factor VIII, and other hemostatic risk factors, may influence this process. CTEPH leads to right ventricular dilatation and dysfunction. The most common symptom during CTEPH is dyspnea due to the development of pulmonary hypertension (PH). In the early stages, dyspnea occurs only during exertion but progressively worsens with the stage and severity of PH. As the disease progresses, symptoms of fatigue, chest pain, syncope, and signs of right heart failure may also occur. The diagnostic algorithm includes evaluating the patient's medical history, signs, and symptoms suggestive of CTEPH, radiological evaluation, lung ventilation-perfusion scintigraphy, and confirmation through hemodynamic evaluation. Ventilation-perfusion lung scintigraphy remains the first-line imaging method for diagnosing CTEPH, offering high sensitivity and specificity for confirming or excluding a diagnosis. While CT pulmonary angiography provides essential information about

* Corresponding Author's Email: esrbinovska@yahoo.com.

In: Pulmonary Embolism
Editors: Irena Mitevska, Sonja Salinger, Marijan Bosevski et al.
ISBN: 979-8-89113-175-0

comorbidities and complications associated with CTEPH, it cannot conclusively rule out a diagnosis. Echocardiography provides comprehensive information on cardiac cavity dimensions, atrial and ventricular function, valvular abnormalities, and assessing hemodynamic parameters related to PH presence. A thorough echocardiographic evaluation for suspected PH includes assessing systolic pulmonary arterial pressure and detecting additional signs suggestive of PH. Pulmonary angiography is the final step in confirming a diagnosis of CTEPH and is an important diagnostic method for evaluating and selecting patients eligible for surgery. Right heart catheterization is also crucial for assessing pressure in the right heart, pulmonary artery, and pulmonary vascular resistance, which are essential long-term prognostic factors in the preoperative and postoperative periods. Distinguishing between CTEPH and idiopathic pulmonary hypertension (IPAH) is critical, as CTEPH can be indicated for endarterectomy and potentially resolved. Balloon pulmonary angioplasty is an emerging treatment modality for inoperable patients, currently limited to experienced and high-volume CTEPH centers.

Keywords: chronic thromboembolic pulmonary hypertension, pulmonary embolism, ventilation-perfusion lung scintigraphy, computed tomography pulmonary angiography, echocardiography

Introduction

Chronic thromboembolic pulmonary hypertension (CTEPH) is classified as group IV in the clinical classification of pulmonary hypertension (PH) according to the new ESC Guidelines for diagnosing and treating pulmonary hypertension. This classification indicates that CTEPH falls under PH associated with pulmonary artery obstructions, either due to chronic thromboembolic pulmonary hypertension or other pulmonary artery obstructions (Table 1) (Humbert et al., 2023).

Pulmonary hypertension is defined by a mean pulmonary pressure (mPAP) greater than 20 mmHg. The latest classification of PH includes pulmonary vascular resistance (PVR) and pulmonary artery wedge pressure (PAWP) in the definition of PH to distinguish elevated PAP due to various causes of pulmonary hypertension. In the case of CTEPH, it leads to pre-capillary hypertension, which is characterized by a combination of mPAP > 20 mmHg, PAWP < 15 mmHg, and PVR > 2 Wood Units (WU). In differentiating between the various causes of pre-capillary, post-capillary, and combined PH, in addition to right ventricular catheterization, the patient's phenotype, risk factors, echocardiographic findings, and other cardiovascular imaging play crucial roles (Humbert et al., 2023).

Table 1. Etiology of PH class IV (Humbert et al., 2022)

Group 4 Pulmonary hypertension
4.1 Chronic thromboembolic pulmonary hypertension (CTEPH)
4.2 Other pulmonary artery obstructions 4.2.1. Sarcoma or angiosarcoma 4.2.2. Other malignant tumors (renal, uterine, germ cell tumor of the testis, other) 4.2.3. Non-malignant tumors (uterine leiomyoma) 4.2.4. Arteritis without connective tissue disease 4.2.5. Congenital pulmonary artery stenosis 4.2.6. Parasites

Pre-capillary hypertension arises from an incomplete resolution of pulmonary embolism (PE) and the formation of a chronic, fibrotic, organized thrombus within the pulmonary vascular bed, which is responsible for reduced or complete obstruction of blood flow (Figure 1) (An et al., 2022; Mahmud et al., 2018).

The incidence of CTEPH is estimated to be 2–6 cases per million adults, and the prevalence is reported to be 26–38 cases per million adults (Delcroix et al., 2020; Kramm et al., 2018; Leber et al., 2021). Patients with CTEPH who do not have PH still comprise a small proportion of those referred to CTEPH centers, represented by patients with chronic thromboembolic diseases (CTED) (Swielik et al., 2019).

CTEPH is a rare but progressive and potentially life-threatening disease that mostly occurs as an uncommon sequel of acute PE, with a cumulative incidence of 0.9–9.1% within 2 years after an acute symptomatic PE, according to prospective observational studies (Humbert et al., 2023; Ruaro et al., 2022). There is variability in the reported occurrence of CTEPH after acute PE due to various factors, including the non-specificity of symptoms and the difficulty distinguishing acute pulmonary embolism from symptoms of pre-existing CTEPH. CTEPH is often under-recognized as its symptomatology depends on the hemodynamic expression of PH (Nishiyama et al., 2018).

According to the international registry, CTEPH is reported to occur in 75% of cases after acute pulmonary thromboembolism, with 56% having a history of documented deep vein thrombosis (Bonderman et al., 2009; Leber et al., 2021; Pepke-Zaba et al., 2011; Simonneau et al., 2022). The most frequent risk factors and predisposing conditions for CTEPH are associated with a diagnosis of pulmonary thromboembolism, documented during the acute phase of PE or within a 3–6-month follow-up period after PE (Table 1 and 2).

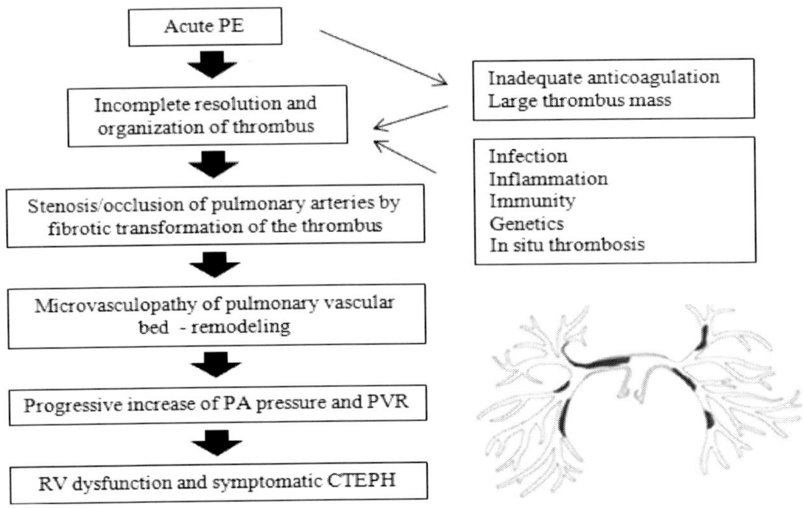

Figure 1. Pathophysiology and natural history of CTEPH (adapted from An J et al., 2022; Lang et al., 2013; Simonneau et al., 2022).

The reason why a certain number of patients develop CTEPH after an acute PE event remains unclear. Table 2 provides the main factors increasing the risk of developing CTEPH after acute PE. These factors include thrombophilic disorders, particularly antiphospholipid antibody syndrome, and elevated coagulation factor VIII levels, as well as conditions like cancer, inflammation, insufficient anticoagulation, splenectomy, and the presence of devices such as implantable pacemakers, among others (Table 2 and Figure 1) (An et al., 2022; Konstantinides et al., 2020; Lang et al., 2013; Simonneau et al., 2022).

Table 2. Predisposing conditions and risk factors for chronic thromboembolic pulmonary hypertension (Konstantinides et al., 2020)

Findings related to the acute PE event (obtained at PE diagnosis)	Concomitant chronic diseases and conditions predisposing to CTEPH (documented at PE diagnosis or at 3–6 month follow-up)
Previous episodes of PE or DVT	Ventriculo-atrial shunts
Large pulmonary arterial thrombi on CTPA	Infected chronic i.v. lines or pacemakers
Echocardiographic signs of PH/RV dysfunction	History of splenectomy
CTPA findings suggestive of pre-existing chronic thromboembolic disease	Thrombophilic disorders, particularly antiphospholipid antibody syndrome and high coagulation factor VIII levels
	Non-O blood group
	Hypothyroidism treated with thyroid hormones
	History of cancer
	Myeloproliferative disorders
	Inflammatory bowel disease
	Chronic osteomyelitis

Pathophysiology and Natural History

CTEPH is considered a rare and late complication of acute PE, persisting for over 3 months despite anticoagulation therapy. In the context of CTEPH, the thrombus undergoes a fibrous transformation in the pulmonary arteries, mechanically obstructing the flow in the affected segment. The presence of organized thrombi in the pulmonary artery segment causes a persistent reduction or obstruction of blood flow, leading to a redistribution of flow across the pulmonary bed and subsequent remodeling of the pulmonary microcirculation. This progressive increase in PVR results in the development of PH (Azarian et al., 1997; Dorfmuller et al., 2014).

Some patients develop CTEPH after an episode of PE while others do not and why the thromboembolic material is replaced by fibrous tissue remains unclear. In most patients with PE, effective mechanisms of endogenous thrombolysis lead to a complete resolution of the thrombus. In some studies, the resolution of the thrombus typically occurs within 30 days after an acute PE, with patients' exercise tolerance completely normalized. A hypothesis suggests that chronic inflammation and ineffective angiogenesis may play a role in the pathogenesis of CTEPH (Quarck et al., 2015).

However, in patients with CTEPH, the process of thrombus resolution after acute PE is ineffective, leading to a reorganization of the thromboembolic material within the vessel wall (Guerin et al., 2014). This process involves thickening the inner layer, forming fibrotic tissue, and developing various degrees of vascular stenosis with forming ring, network, or band-like structures that obstruct blood flow. These changes increase vascular resistance and pulmonary arterial pressure.

The pathophysiology of CTEPH is complex, and much remains to be clarified. Increasing evidence suggests that CTEPH is not solely attributed to chronic mechanical obstruction from residual thrombotic material but also involves remodeling and microvasculopathy of the distal pulmonary arteries. Various pathological changes in small blood vessels have been observed in patients with CTEPH and those exhibiting distal perfusion defects. These changes include obstruction of small elastic sub-segmental arteries, intimal thickening of blood vessels, and hypertrophy of the muscular layer in small arteries and arterioles. Interestingly, the described changes bear similarities to the vascular lesions observed in patients with idiopathic pulmonary arterial hypertension (Guerin et al., 2015; Ruaro et al., 2022).

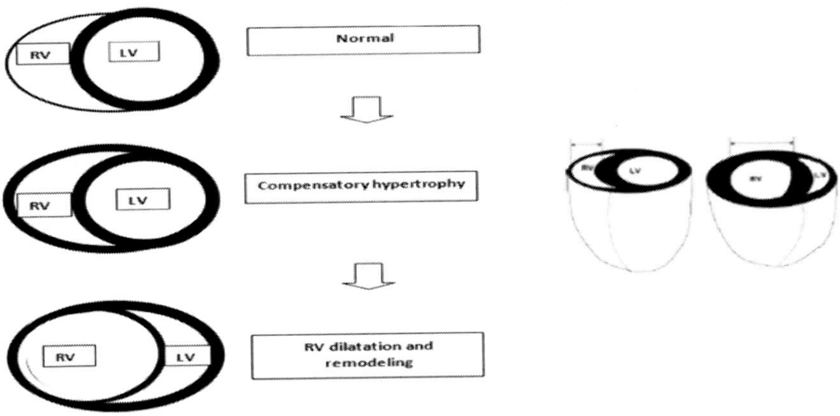

Figure 2. Right ventricular remodeling in patients with CTEPH.

The geometry of the right ventricle (RV) is highly complex, with its wall being thinner than that of the left ventricle (LV). In the case of CTEPH, significant morphological and functional adaptive changes occur in the RV. The initial adaptation is RV myocardial hypertrophy, which can lead to progressive dilation, remodeling, and impaired contractility of the RV, resulting in RV dysfunction (Figure 2). The dilation of the RV also leads to tricuspid annular dilation and functional tricuspid regurgitation. As hypertrophy and dilation progress, the RV assumes a more spherical shape, its cross-sectional area enlarges, and the interventricular septum flattens, causing impaired filling of the LV. This can decrease stroke volume (Badano et al., 2010; Humbert et al., 2022; Rudski et al., 2010).

Clinical Presentation and Diagnosis

Clinical Presentation

CTEPH primarily affects adults, with an average age of 63 years, and there is no significant difference between genders. Early detection of CTEPH is challenging and often takes an average of 14 months from the onset of symptoms in expert centers. Patients may remain completely asymptomatic during the disease development phase, often called the "honeymoon period," following an embolic event. The symptomatology is non-specific and becomes evident as right heart failure and PH progressively develop, which is characteristic of the advanced stages of the disease (Konstantinides et al., 2020; Ruaro et al., 2022).

Patients with complete unilateral obstruction may exhibit normal pulmonary hemodynamics at rest despite having symptomatic disease, and they are classified as having CTED (Lung et al., 2021). Post-PE syndrome is defined as persistent dyspnea, impaired exercise capacity, and/or decreased health-related quality of life (Simonneau et al., 2023).

The persistent reduction or obstruction of the pulmonary arteries in CTEPH leads to the development of PH, which in turn causes right ventricular dilatation and dysfunction. During the early stages of PH development, clinical symptoms are often associated with dyspnea on exertion, fatigue, palpitations, chronic nonproductive cough, and sometimes atypical chest pain. Dyspnea is classified according to the World Health Organization Functional Class (WHO-FC) system. As the disease progresses, dyspnea worsens, occurring with even less effort, and this progression correlates with the stage and severity of the disease. In the later stages of the disease, signs of RV dysfunction and PH become more evident, such as weight gain due to fluid retention, hemoptysis, and syncope during or shortly after physical exertion

(Humbert et al., 2023). Clinical deterioration is typically associated with impaired RV function. The 6-minute walking test is commonly used to provide prognostic information in patients with CTEPH (Miller et al., 2022; Nishiyama et al., 2018).

Certain electrocardiogram abnormalities, such as P pulmonale, right or sagittal axis deviation, and signs of right ventricular hypertrophy or right bundle branch block, may raise suspicion of PH and the development of CTEPH (Figure 3).

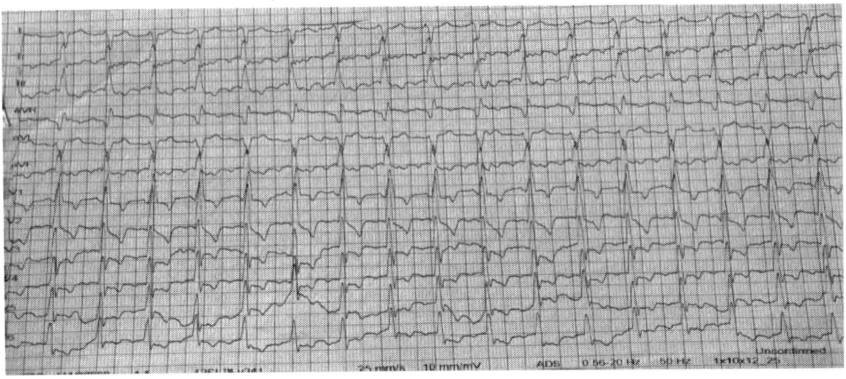

Figure 3. ECG in a patient with CTEPH.

Some ECG abnormalities in clinically suspected PH, particularly in cases of unexplained dyspnea on exertion, have a high predictive value for PH (Kovacs et al., 2016; Henkens et al., 2008). A normal ECG does not completely rule out the presence of PH, but a normal ECG combined with normal biomarkers (BNP/NT-proBNP) is associated with a low likelihood of PH in patients suspected of or at risk for PH, such as after acute PE (Bonderman et al., 2011; Klok et al., 2011; Morris et al., 2022).

Diagnosis of CTEPH

CTEPH is a significant cause of PH with a distinct management strategy. Timely diagnosis of CTEPH is crucial for referring patients to specialized CTEPH/PH centers and selecting the appropriate treatment strategy.

The diagnosis of CTEPH is based on evidence of pre-capillary PH assessed by right heart catheterization (RHC), along with at least one segmental perfusion defect evident on V/Q scan and other modalities for perfusion (computed tomography pulmonary angiography (CTPA), cardiac magnetic resonance (CMR), and pulmonary angiography (PA). Additionally, signs of chronic thromboembolism visible on CTPA angiography or pulmonary angiography (annular stenosis, chronic lesions, and/or complete occlusions) are considered in the diagnostic process. The diagnostic algorithm should also include an evaluation of the patient's medical history and signs and symptoms suggestive of CTEPH, especially in patients who have undergone effective anticoagulation therapy for at least 3 months after an episode of PE or have other risk factors predisposing to CTEPH (Humbert et al., 2023) (Figure 4, Table 3).

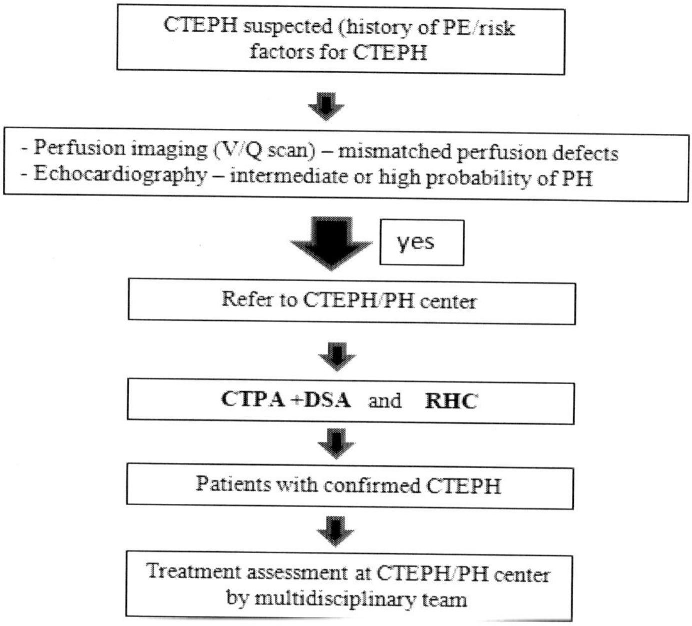

Figure 4. Diagnostic algorithm in patients with CTEPH (Adapted from Humbert et al., 2023).

Multidisciplinary CTEPH teams are mandatory for providing complex multimodal treatment recommendations and individual long-term follow-up and therapy (Simonnneau et al., 2023). Diagnostic delay in patients with CTEPH is associated with a poor outcomes, lower quality of life, and a higher risk of death. A large RV diameter with an RV/LV ratio greater than 1, high pulmonary arterial pressure, and RV dysfunction were identified as independent predictors of impending CTEPH (An et al., 2022; Bossone et al., 2013).

Table 3. Clinical and diagnostics characteristics of CTEPH (adapted by Lang et al., 2021)

Clinical and diagnostic criteria	CTEPH
Symptoms	Exercise and resting dyspnea
V/Q scan	Mismatched ventilation/perfusion defects
CTPA or DSA	Ring-like stenosis, webs/slits and chronic total occlusion
TTE	Enlarged RA and RV or normal, PH present or absent
RHC	mPAP>25mmHg, PAWP <15mmHg
Anticoagulation before diagnosis	At least 3 months

V/Q scan – ventilation-perfusion scintigraphy; CTPA – computed tomography pulmonary angiography; DSA – digital subtraction angiography; TTE – transthoracic echocardiography, RA – right atrium; RV – right ventricle; PH – pulmonary hypertension; RHC – right heart catheterization, mPAP – mean pressure in the pulmonary artery, PA WP – pulmonary artery wedge pressure.

The diagnostic modalities should aim to establish a differential diagnosis for CTEPH and exclude conditions such as IPAH, pulmonary arteritis, pulmonary angiosarcoma, tumor embolism, parasites (hydatid cyst), foreign body embolism, and congenital or acquired PA stenosis (Konstadinidies et al., 2020).

Ventilation/Perfusion Scintigraphy

According to current guidelines, a ventilation/perfusion (V/Q) scan is recommended as the first-line imaging modality for CTEPH, with a sensitivity of 96-97% and specificity of 90-95% for diagnosis. V/Q scan is one of the most useful imaging modalities for screening CTEPH, as it can reveal at least one segmental perfusion defect despite normal ventilation. Additionally, the V/Q scan is valuable in discriminating CTEPH from acute PE (Figure 5) (Konstantinides et al., 2014; Kim et al., 2023; Nishiyama et al., 2018).

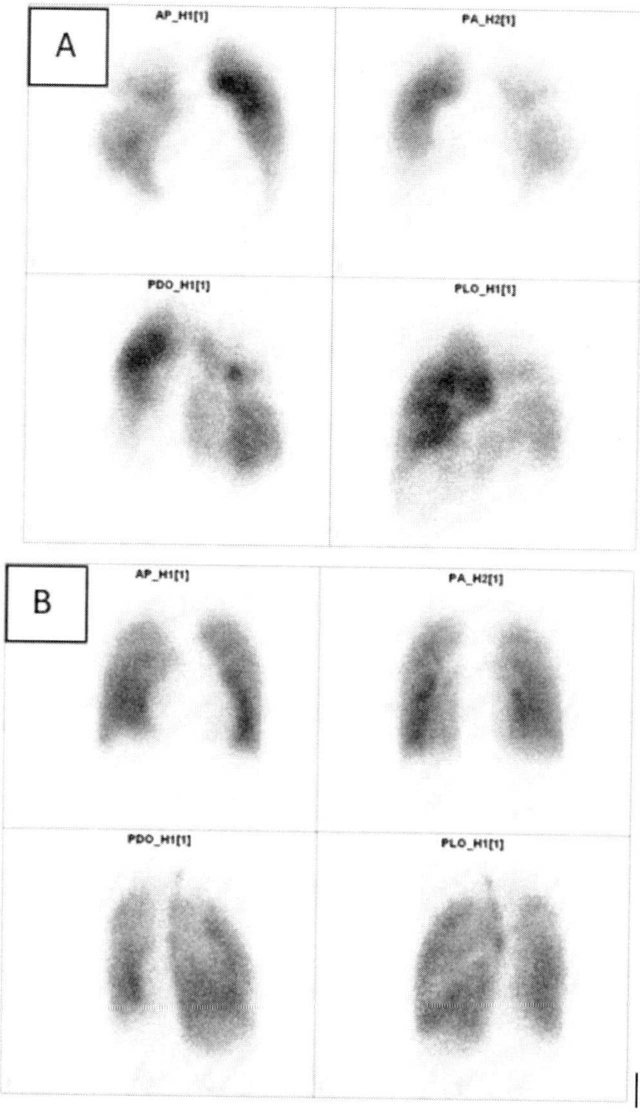

Figure 5. (A) Lung planar perfusion scan with 99mTc MAA (Q-study) in standard scan positions (AP, PA, DPO, LPO) with multiple segmental and sub-segmental perfusion outbursts in both lungs, with a characteristic wedge shape and extension of the base to the pleura, highly suspicious for massive pulmonary thromboembolism; (B) Lung planar ventilation scan with 99mTc DTPA (V-study), in standard scan positions (AP, PA, DPO, LPO)shows orderly, homogeneous ventilation of all lung segments(regular ventilation in the segments with perfusion outbursts) The combined V/Q-study points to a mismatch of ventilation and perfusion findings.

Normal findings on the V/Q scan usually exclude the presence of CTEPH. However, false-negative results may occur due to the recanalization of chronic thrombi, or false interpretations can be attributed to chronic hypo perfusion of the lungs, leading to decreased ventilation. In cases of high probability and non-diagnostic scans, further diagnostic investigations, primarily perfusion imaging modalities, are required. Single-photon emission computed tomography (SPECT) can enhance accuracy in detecting and quantifying perfusion defects compared to planar V/Q scans. Other causes of PH typically present with normal scans or non-segmental perfusion abnormalities. V/Q scan is a safer choice for diagnosis than CTPA in patients with severe iodine contrast allergy and reduced renal function (Nishiyama et al., 2018; Simonneau et al., 2023).

Computed Tomography Pulmonary Angiography

Recent evidence suggests that the diagnostic performance of CTPA in CTEPH is non-inferior to that of a V/Q scan. Studies have demonstrated high specificity and sensitivity of CTPA for detecting CTED at the lobar level (97–100% sensitivity and 95–100% specificity) and segmental level (86–100% sensitivity and 93–99% specificity). However, a negative CTPA does not completely rule out CTEPH, especially in cases of CTEPH at the sub-segmental level (Nishiyama KH et al., 2018; Konstantinides SV et al., 2020).

CTPA can typically distinguish between acute and chronic pulmonary thromboembolism. In cases of chronic pulmonary thromboembolism, there may be partial obstruction, identified as a partially attenuated vessel, or dilatation distal to the obstruction with a narrow diameter. Complete obstruction of the blood vessel manifests as a lack of contrast distal to the site of obstruction (Poor H et al., 2023). An important specific finding of CTEPH on CTPA is the presence of eccentric wall-adherent or mural thrombi, which are often calcified. Complete vessel cutoff with a convex margin due to organized thrombi is another distinct feature of CTEPH, differentiating it from the concave margin observed in acute PE with a tapering thrombus. Additionally, an abrupt narrowing of the vessel distal to complete obstruction is a common finding in CTEPH, resulting from the contraction of the thrombus, and the development of collateral systemic circulation, such as bronchial artery dilatation, is frequently observed. Furthermore, non-uniform arterial perfusion patterns and a mosaic pattern of lung attenuation can be observed (Bryce et al., 2019; Kim et al., 2021).

In CTEPH, in addition to the vascular signs present on CTPA, there may also be signs in favor of PH, such as main PA dilatation with usually asymmetric dilatation of the PA branches, an enlarged RV, RV hypertrophy, and an RV/LV diameter ratio greater than 1. Additionally, bowing of the interventricular septum toward the LV may be observed. Lung parenchymal signs in CTEPH can include scars from prior pulmonary infarctions (e.g., parenchymal bands, irregular peripheral linear opacities, and wedge-shaped opacities with pleural thickening) and mosaic lung attenuation due to heterogeneous perfusion. It's important to note that mosaic lung attenuation is non-specific and can also be seen in patients with PH due to cardiac or lung diseases (Figures 6 and 7) (Nishiyama et al., 2018; Simonneau et al., 2023).

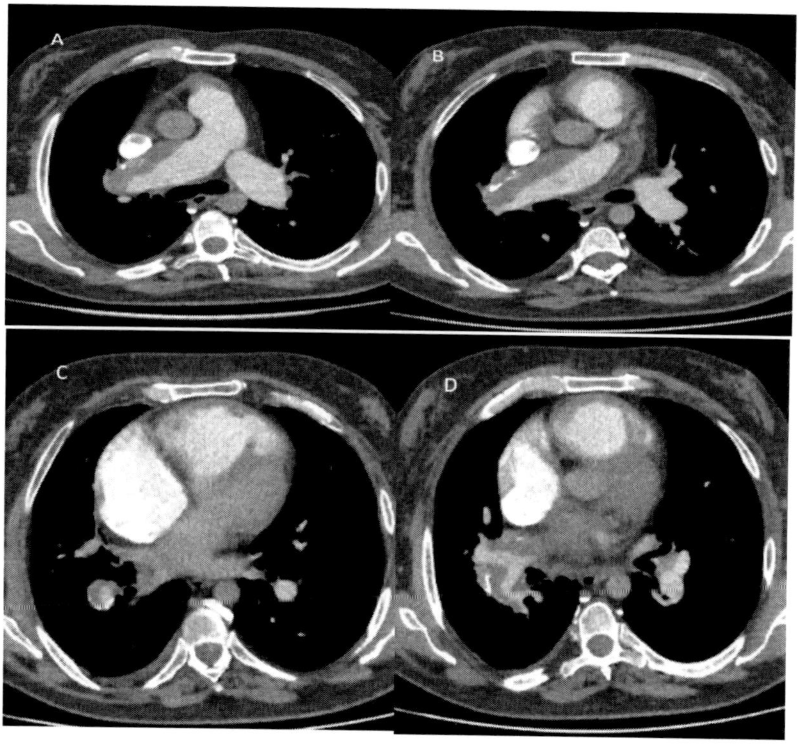

Figure 6. CTPA in patients with CTEPH. (A and B). Extensive peripheral thromboembolic filling defects in the right pulmonary artery; (C) Peripheral thromboembolic filling defects at the level of the bifurcation of the right lobar arteries for the middle and lower lobe; (D). Chronic thromboembolic changes in the right lower lobe artery with small pleural effusion.

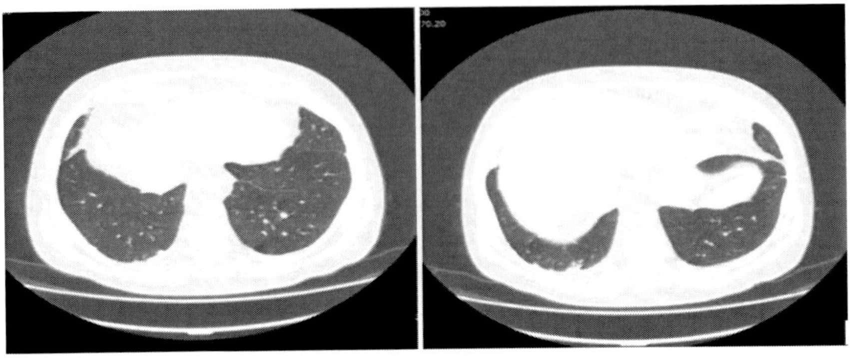

Figure 7. CTPA in patients with CTEPH. Sub-pleural condensations in the lung parenchyma postero-basally on the right in addition to ischemic lung changes.

Despite CTPA gaining ground as a diagnostic modality in CTEPH, it should not be used as a stand-alone test to exclude the disease (Konstantinides et al., 2020).

Dual-energy CT (DECT) angiography and iodine subtraction mapping may provide additional diagnostic information for lung perfusion, thereby possibly increasing the diagnostic accuracy for CTEPH. DECT allows the simultaneous assessment of the patency of the PA and lung perfusion (Humbert et al., 2023; Konstantinides et al., 2020).

Digital subtraction angiography (DSA) is mainly used to confirm the diagnosis of CTEPH and to assess treatment options (pulmonary endarterectomy (PEA) or balloon pulmonary angioplasty (BPA)) (Humbert et al., 2023).

Echocardiography

Echocardiography is widely used as the initial diagnostic tool when suspected PH. Routine echocardiography at 6 weeks after PE has been suggested to identify patients at risk for developing CTEPH (Hoeper et al., 2006). However, an indication for echocardiography exists whenever there are symptoms after acute PE.

Transthoracic comprehensive echocardiography (TEE) with all echocardiographic modalities can provide useful information about the hemodynamic changes in the RV and LV that occur in CTEPH, as shown in Figures 8 and 9. TEE can detect and evaluate PH and PVR through the maximum velocity of tricuspid regurgitation and other signs suggesting PH, as shown in Tables 4 and 5. In the early phase of PH, with the increasing afterload, the RV undergoes initial adaptation with RV hypertrophy and an increase in the mass of the RV, representing adaptive remodeling. As the disease progresses, the hypertrophic process may slow down, and RV dilatation begins to progress.

In the new Guidelines on Diagnosis and Treatment of PH, all echocardiographic features that can be evaluated by echocardiography are provided (Humbert et al., 2023). Figure 9 illustrates a large RV with hypertrophy, RV/LV ratio greater than 1, eccentricity index larger than 1, D-shape of the LV with small LV end-diastolic dimension due to RV overload, and dilated non-collapsible inferior vena cava (Chapter 4).

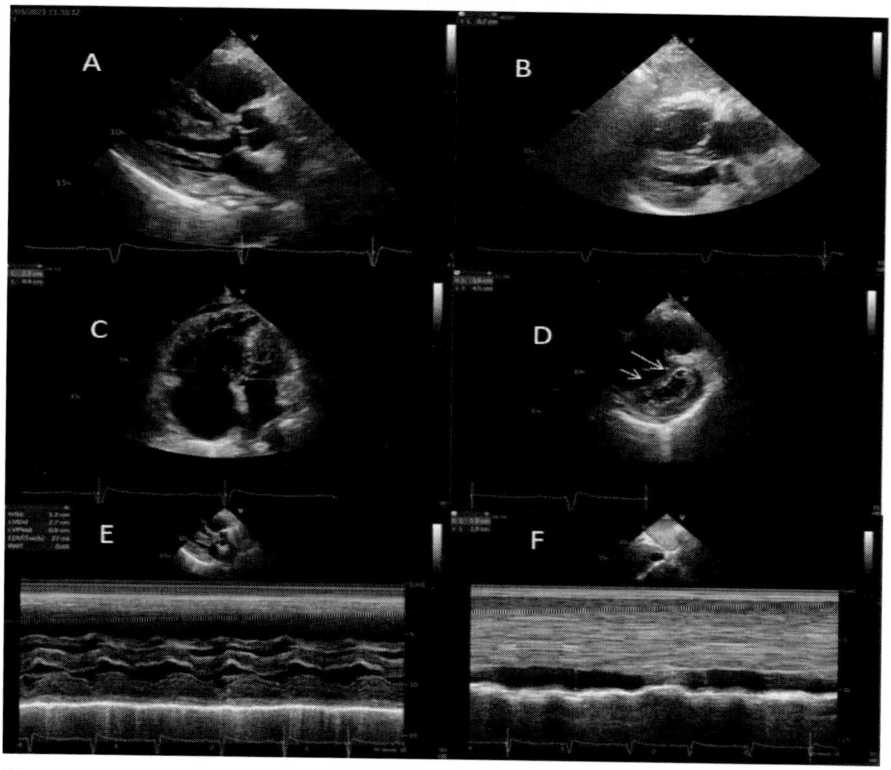

Figure 8. Two-dimensional transthoracic echocardiography in patent with CTEPH (A) PLAX – small LV and large RV with hypertrophy of the RV structures and RV wall; (B) Sub-costal view – RV hypertrophy (7 mm); (C) Four-chamber view - RV/LV ration bigger than 1; (D) Short axis of the left ventricle on the papillary level -D-shape of the LV, eccentricity index bigger than 1; (E) M-mode of the LV – small LV end-diastolic dimension due to RV overload; (F). Sub-costal view – dilated vena cava inferior, with non-collapsibility of more than 50%.

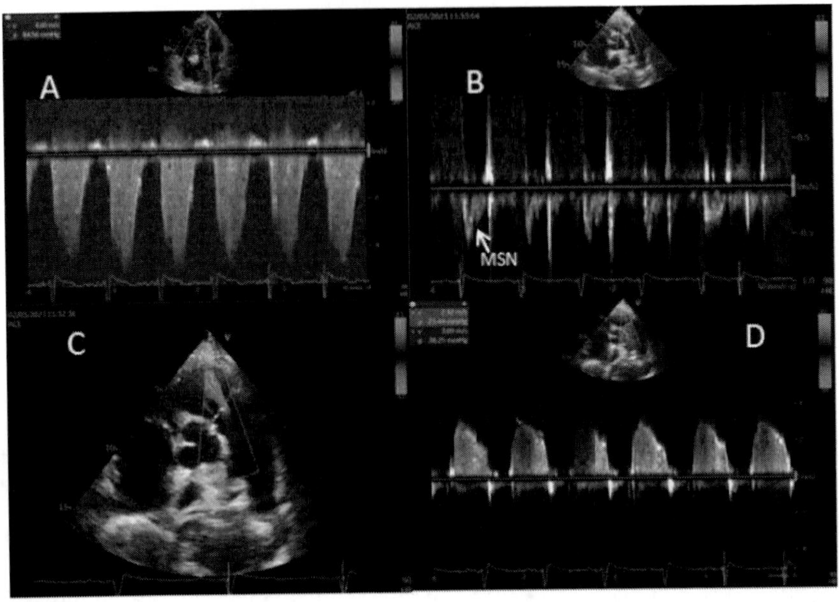

Figure 9. Two-dimensional transthoracic echocardiography in patent with CTEPH (A) Continuous Doppler of tricuspid regurgitation showing very high peak velocity of tricuspid regurgitation (V of TR- 4.8 m/s); (B) Pulsed Doppler on right outflow tract, before pulmonary artery showing shortened acceleration time of and present of mid systolic notch (MSN); (C and D) Dilated pulmonary artery and branches with severe pulmonary regurgitation on short axis on the base of the heart and continuous Doppler record.

Estimating the systolic PA pressure (sPAP) is based on the peak velocity of the tricuspid regurgitation jet. PH is estimated from the peak velocity of the tricuspid regurgitation using a simplified Bernoulli equation.

sPAP (mmHg) = 4(V max of the TR)2+RAP, where V is velocity, TR – tricuspid regurgitation, and RAP is right atrial pressure.

Severe TR is associated with a low jet velocity due to the reduced transvalvular gradient between the right atrium (RA) and right ventricle (RV), which can lead to an underestimation of PH. Additionally, the Bernoulli equation can be used to estimate mean pulmonary pressure (mean PAP) and diastolic pulmonary pressure (dPAP) based on the velocity of the pulmonary regurgitation (PR) velocity, measured from the peak velocity at the beginning and the end of the diastolic flow (Figure 10). Estimating PH based on Doppler echocardiography is unsuitable for mild, asymptomatic PH (Srbinovska E.,

2013). Additional echocardiographic parameters should be considered to diagnose possible PH (Tables 4 and 5).

Several echocardiographic parameters are important for the estimation and follow-up of right ventricular function, such as RA and RV dimensions and volumes, functional area changes, D-shape of the LV, tricuspid annular plane systolic excursion (TAPSE), myocardial performance index, inferior vena cava dimensions and collapsibility, S velocity estimated by Tissue Doppler Imaging, and global strain of the RV (Figure 10) (Jones et al., 2019; Humbert et al., 2023; Lang et al., 2015).

Table 4. Echocardiographic probability of PH in symptomatic patients suspected of PH (Galie et al., 2016)

Peak TR velocity (m/s)	Presence of other echo PH signs	Echocardiographic probability of PH
<2/8 or not measurable	No	Low
<2.8 or not measurable	Yes	Intermediate
2.9-3.4	No	Intermediate
2.9-3.4	Yes	High
>3.4	Not require	High

Table 5. Echocardiographic signs suggesting PH are used to assess the probability of PH in addition to TR velocity measurement (Galie et al., 2016, Humbert et al., 2023)

The ventricle	Pulmonary artery (PA)	Inferior vena cava (IVC) and right atrium (RA)
RV/LV basal diameter >1.0	RVOT AT <105 ms and or MSN	IVC>21 with decreased inspiratory collapse (<50% with a sniff of <20% with quiet inspiration)
Flattening of the interventricular septum	Early diastolic pulmonary regurgitation velocity >2.2 m/s	RA area (end-systole) >18 cm^2
TAPSE/sPAP ratio <0.55 mm/mmHg	PA diameter > aortic root diameter PA diameter >25 mm	

Abbreviations: RV-right ventricle; LV- left ventricle; RVOT- right ventricular outflow tract; AT = acceleration time; IVC- inferior vena cava; RA- right atrium; PA - pulmonary artery; TAPSE- tricuspid annular plane systolic excursion.

Several echocardiographic parameters have been established as important for predicting the prognosis of the disease. Patients with PH who develop RV dysfunction tend to experience a poor quality of life and have a worse outcome.

Reverse remodeling, characterized by a reduction in RV mass and volume, has been associated with successful interventions through pharmacological treatments, pulmonary endarterectomy, or balloon dilatation. Echocardiographic evidence of reverse RV remodeling has been shown to be a stronger prognostic indicator than functional and hemodynamic parameters.

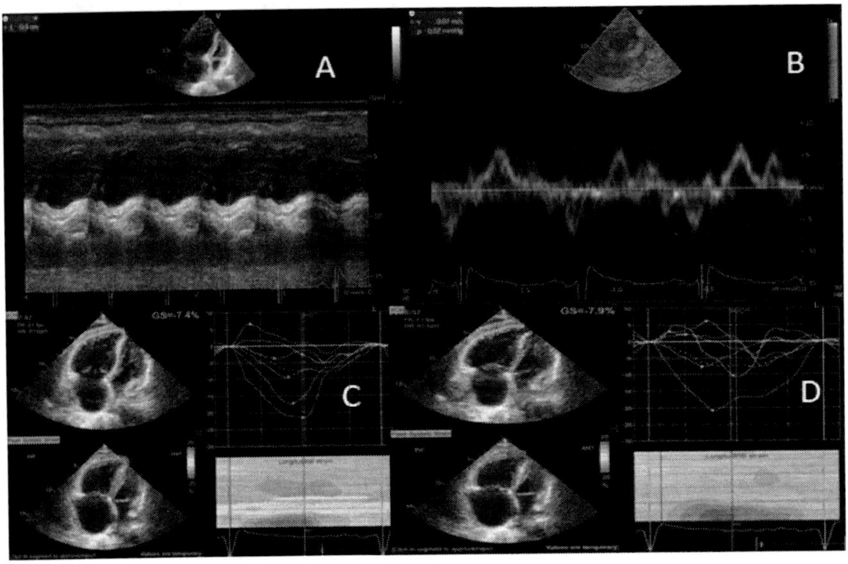

Figure 10. Two-dimensional transthoracic echocardiography in patent with CTEPH (A) M-mode placed on four-chamber view showing reduced tricuspid annular plane systolic excursion (TAPSE) - 13 mm; (B) Tissue Doppler recording under tricuspid annulus showing reduced systolic velocity – 0.07m/s; (C and D) Global longitudinal strain (GLS) of the right ventricle and on the free wall of the right ventricle showing reduction of GLS -7.4% and -7.9%.

Magnetic Resonance Pulmonary Angiography

Magnetic resonance imaging (MRI) in patients with CTEPH allows for assessing the pulmonary arterial circulation, evaluating pulmonary perfusion, and accurate and reproducible functional assessment of RV dysfunction and hypertrophy, as well as the hemodynamic impact of cardiac function. Magnetic resonance pulmonary angiography (MRPA) has a sensitivity of 97%, specificity of 92%, positive predictive value of 95%, and negative predictive value of 96% for detecting CTEPH. MRPA can recognize irregular luminal filling defects, intraluminal webs and bands, vessel cutoffs, and organized thrombi. However, MRI imaging is still considered inferior to CT in assessing pulmonary vasculature. A disadvantage of the method is its relatively longer scan time, relatively lower spatial resolution, and limited parenchymal evaluation (Konstantinides et al., 2020; Kreitner et al., 2004; Nishiyama et al., 2018).

Right Heart Catheterization and Pulmonary Angiography

After non-invasive imaging modalities, it is necessary to perform RHC to assess the severity of hemodynamic impairment and confirm the diagnosis of CTEPH. RHC is fundamental for diagnosing CTEPH, as it allows for the direct determination of mPAP and PAWP and provides information on disease severity, right heart function, and mixed venous oxygen saturation. RHC is also used to guide treatment decisions and assess surgical eligibility. The procedure requires meticulous attention to detail and should be limited to expert centers to obtain high-quality results. RHC is also utilized to perform pulmonary angiography (PA).

Pulmonary angiography is more useful in patients suspected of having CTEPH, as it can help recognize complete vessel cutoff with the convex contour of thrombi, abrupt vessel narrowing, luminal irregularities, and intravascular bands or webs. A correct differential diagnosis between CTEPH and idiopathic pulmonary hypertension (IPAH) is essential to make a therapeutic decision since CTEPH can potentially be resolved by endarterectomy (Ruaro et al., 2022).

Treatment and Prognosis

CTEPH is often underdiagnosed, and its prognosis is poor if left untreated. The importance of timely and accurate diagnosis for CTEPH lies in the fact that it is the only type of PH potentially curable through pulmonary endarterectomy (PEA) surgery. Multidisciplinary CTEPH teams are essential for providing complex multimodal treatment recommendations and individual long-term follow-up and therapy. Medical therapy and balloon pulmonary angioplasty (BPA) have provided alternative therapeutic options for patients with inoperable CTEPH. Treatment modalities are available for each compartment of the affected PA: PEA for proximal vessels, BPA for distal vessels, and PH drugs for microcirculation (Simonneau et al., 2023).

Echocardiographic findings can be an important guide for managing and following up patients with CTEPH and evaluating patients post-treatment (PEA or BPA) and reversal remodeling.

Pulmonary Endarterectomy

Pulmonary endarterectomy is the treatment of choice, which can significantly improve the quality of life. Pharmacological treatment and balloon angioplasty should be offered to patients who are not candidates for surgery or have recurrent pulmonary embolism despite PEA.

PEA is the treatment of choice in patients who are considered operative candidates and have obstructing lesions in the main, lobar, segmental, and sub-segmental arteries (Figure 11). The procedure involves the removal of the obstructive thromboembolic material from the vessel wall. The surgical approach requires a median sternotomy and the use of a heart-lung machine with deep hypothermia and circulatory arrest. The hemodynamic results after PEA are immediately evident, with a return in most cases to normal values. After a few days, there is an initial recovery of cardiac function with a reduction of RV dilatation, and after one year, there is reverse remodeling of the RV with the disappearance of RV hypertrophy, as well as normalization of ventricular wall movement. The functional improvement occurs gradually and, above all, depends on the patient's age and disease duration (Ahn et al., 2019; Ruaro et al., 2022).

Intra and peri-operative complications of PEA are frequent, such as lung perfusion injury and hemoptysis, which can usually be managed conservatively. However, in 2–3% of patients, the bleeding rate and parenchymal edema can be severe and cause life-threatening hypoxemia. Residual PH with RV failure is less common, which is a result of a poor surgical outcome. The hospital mortality of PEA depends on the degree of experience of the center and is about 3.5% in specialized centers. Additionally, hospital mortality is influenced by PVR and the type of thromboembolic lesions (Cullivan et al., 2023; Ruaro et al., 2022).

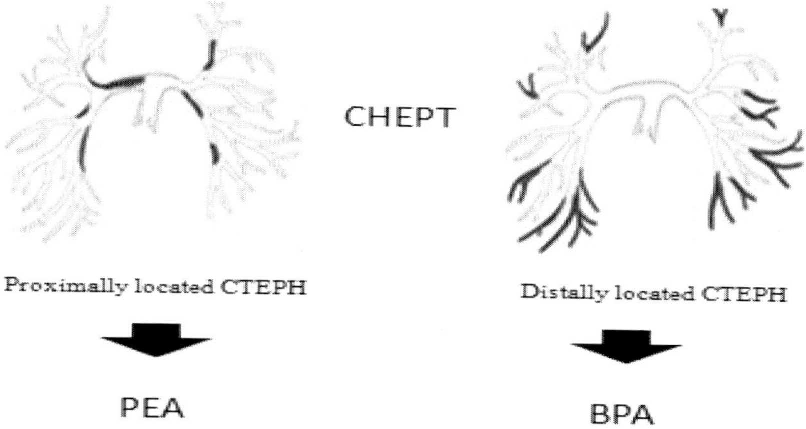

Figure 11. Schema for CTEPH management (adapted from An et al., 2022).

Balloon Pulmonary Angioplasty

BPA is an effective alternative therapy for patients with inoperable CTEPH. It is a stepwise procedure requiring several separate sessions, typically 4-10, which allows for the dilatation of obstructions down to sub-segmental lesions inaccessible to surgery. Due to the complexity and individual variability of the pulmonary arterial tree, the procedure requires an experienced team and expertise. Several types of lesions have been described: type A - ring-like stenosis lesion; type B - web lesion; type C - subtotal lesion; type D - total occlusion lesion; and type E - tortuous lesion (Kawakami et al., 2016). The success rate was higher, and the complication rate was lower in ring-like stenosis and web lesions. Total occlusion lesions had the lowest success rate, and tortuous lesions had a high complication rate. Complications can include wire and balloon-induced injury, which may result in intrapulmonary bleeding, hemoptysis, and reperfusion lung injury.

Published data have shown significant improvements in functional class and a significant reduction in the average pulmonary arterial pressure from 45 to 24 mmHg with BPA. BPA-associated mortality ranged from 0% to 3.4%, and BPA-related lung injury occurred in 9% to 60% of cases. A lower incidence of serious adverse events related to BPA was reported when patients received a 26-week treatment with riociguat prior to BPA, optimizing pre-BPA hemodynamics. BPA has also been used as a sequential treatment for PH persisting after PEA (Delcroix et al., 2016; Konstantinides et al., 2020; Mizoguchi et al., 2012; Ruaro et al., 2022).

Pharmacological Treatment

Pharmacological treatment in patients with CTEPH remains insufficiently defined and challenging. The optimal medical approach for CTEPH involves lifelong oral anticoagulants as the mainstay therapy and symptomatic management using diuretics and oxygen when necessary for heart failure, PH, and hypoxemia. Lifelong oral vitamin K antagonist (VKA) therapy is recommended for patients with CTEPH and also for those who have undergone successful pulmonary endarterectomy (PEA) or BPA. While increasing evidence supports the safety of direct oral anticoagulants (DOACs) as an alternative to VKAs, data on their efficacy and safety in CTEPH patients are still lacking.

Comparable findings from the EXPERT registry have shown that the rate of recurrent venous thromboembolism (VTE) was higher in patients receiving DOACs than those receiving VKAs, though the rate of bleeding events was similar between the two groups. VKAs are specifically indicated in cases of antiphospholipid syndrome, which may be present in up to 10% of patients with CTEPH. The primary goal of anticoagulant therapy is to prevent thrombosis within the pulmonary arteries and episodes of VTE (Humbert et al., 2022; Konstantinides et al., 2020; Simonneau et al., 2015).

Regarding therapy for PH and microvasculopathy, the only drug registered and approved for inoperable CTEPH or persistent/recurrent PH after pulmonary endarterectomy (PEA) is riociguat, an oral stimulator of soluble guanylate cyclase. Treatment with riociguat has significantly increased the 6-minute walking distance and reduced PVR. In contrast, patients treated with bosentan only demonstrated hemodynamic improvement. Currently, riociguat is recommended as bridging therapy for patients scheduled to undergo PEA (Konstantinides et al., 2020; Cullivan et al., 2023). Additionally, treprostinil has shown efficacy in treating CTEPH, and macitentan at higher doses is currently under investigation.

The optimal use and benefits of many therapies remain unclear, and there is often a poor correlation between hemodynamic and functional outcomes, highlighting the necessity for further controlled trials.

Conclusion

CTEPH is characterized by persistent PA obstruction due to chronic organized fibrotic clots, even with adequate anticoagulation. These pathophysiological changes lead to pre-capillary hypertension, often accompanied by microvasculopathy. Over time, PH can result in progressive right heart failure, which can be assessed through echocardiography. The combination of persistent dyspnea, exercise intolerance, and reduced quality of life necessitates diagnostic procedures to confirm or exclude CTEPH, especially if dyspnea persists for more than 3 months after confirmed PE. Diagnostic delays are associated with poorer outcomes, lower quality of life, and increased risk of death. Timely and accurate diagnosis requires a combination of imaging and hemodynamic assessments in patients suspected of having CTEPH.

V/Q scintigraphy remains the standard method to rule out chronic thromboembolism, but there is growing evidence supporting perfusion CT and MR perfusion as diagnostic tools for CTEPH. RHC and CT pulmonary angiography (CTPA) are the gold standards for assessing operability. Multidisciplinary CTEPH teams are essential for providing complex multimodal treatment recommendations and individual long-term follow-up and therapy.

Anticoagulant therapy is indicated in almost all patients with CTEPH, depending on the underlying pathogenesis. Riociguat (an oral soluble guanylate cyclase stimulator) has become the first approved treatment for patients with inoperable disease or recurrent PE. Pulmonary endarterectomy is the treatment of choice for improving quality of life. Pharmacological treatment and balloon angioplasty should be considered for patients who are unsuitable for surgery or who experience recurrent pulmonary embolism despite PEA.

References

Ahn, C., and Hiromi, M.: Chronic thromboembolic pulmonary hypertension: endovascular treatment; *Korean Circ J.* 2019; 49(3):214-222.

An, J., Nam, Y., Cho, H., Chang, J., Kim, D. K., and Lee, K. S. Acute Pulmonary Embolism and Chronic Tromboembolic Pulmonary Hypertension: Clinical and Serial CT Pulmonary Angiographic Features. *J. Korean Med. Sci.,* (2022)37(10):e76.

Azarian, R., Wartski, M., Collignon, M. A., Parent, F., Herve, P., Sors, H., Simonneau, G.: Lung perfusion scans and hemodynamics in acute and chronic pulmonary embolism. *J Nucl Med* 1997;38:980-983.

Badano, L., Ginghina, C., Easaw, J., Muraru, D., Grillo, M. T., Lancellotti, P., Pinamonti, B., Coghlan, G., Marra, M. P., Popescu, B. A., De Vita, S. Right ventricle in pulmonary arterial hypertension: haemodynamics, structural changes, imaging and proposal of a study protocol aimed to assess remodeling and treatment effects; *Eur J of Echocardiography* (2010):11, 27-37.

Bonderman, D., Wexberg, P., Martischnig, A. M., Heinzl, H., Lang, M. B., Sadushi, R, Skoro-Sajer, N., Lang, I. M. A non-invasive algorithm to exclude pre-capillary pulmonary hypertension. *Eur Respir J* 2011;37:1096–1103.

Bonderman, D., Wilkens, H., Wakounig, S., Schafers, H. J., Jansa, P., Lindner, J., Simkova, I., Martischnig, A. M., Dudczak, J., Sadushi, R., Skoro-Sajer, N., Klepetko, W., Lang, I. M. Risk factors for chronic thromboembolic pulmonary hypertension. *Eur Respir J* 2009;33:325_331.

Bossone, E., D'Andrea, A., D'Alto, M., Citro, R., Argiento, P., Ferrara, F., Cittadini, A., Rubenfire, M., Naeije, R. Echocardiography in Pulmonary arterial Hypertension: from Diagnosis to Prognosis, State of the art review article; *Journal of the American Society of Echocardiography*, Vol. 26, No.1,2013.

Bryce, Y. C., Perez-Johnston, R., Bryce, E. B., Homayoon, B., Santos-Martin, E. G., Pathophisiology of right ventricular failure in acute pulmonary embolism and chronic tromboembolic pulmonary hypertension: a pictorial essay for the interventional radiologist; *Insights into imaging* (2019) 10:18.

Cullivan, S., Gaine, S., Sitbon, O.: New trends in pulmonary hypertension. *Eur Respir Rev* 2023;32:220211.

Delcroix, M., Lang, I., Pepke-Zaba, J., Jansa, P., D'Armini, A. M., Snijder, R., Bresser, P., Torbicki, A., Mellemkjaer, S., Lewczuk, J., Simkova, I., Barberà, J. A., de Perrot, M., Hoeper, M.M., Gaine, S., Speich, R., Gomez-Sanchez, M. A., Kovacs, G., Jaïs, X., Ambroz, D., Treacy, C., Morsolini, M., Jenkins, D., Lindner, J., Dartevelle, P., Mayer, E., Simonneau, G.. Long-term outcome of patients with chronic thromboembolic pulmonary hypertension: Results from an international prospective registry. *Circulation* 2016, 133, 859–871.

Dorfmuller, P., Gunther, S., Ghigna, M.R., de Montpreville V.T., Boulate, D., Paul, J. F., Jais, X., Decante, B., Simonneau, G., Dartevelle, P., Humbert, M., Fadel, E., Mercier, O. Microvascular disease in chronic thromboembolic pulmonary hypertension: a role for pulmonary veins and systemic vasculature. *Eur Respir J* 2014;44:1275-1288.

Galiè, N., Humbert, M., Vachiery, J. V., Gibbs, S., Lang, I., Torbicki, A., Simonneau, G., Peacock, A., Noordegraaf, A. V., Beghetti, M., Ghofrani, M. A., Sanchez, M. A., Hansmann, G., Klepetko, W., Lancellotti, P., Matucci, M., McDonagh, T., Pierard, L. A., Trindade, P. T., Zompatori, M., Hoeper, M., ESC Scientific Document Group. 2015 ESC/ERS Guidelines for the diagnosis and treatment of pulmonary hypertension: The Joint Task Force for the Diagnosis and Treatment of Pulmonary Hypertension of the European Society of Cardiology (ESC) and the European Respiratory Society (ERS): Endorsed by: Association for European Paediatric and Congenital Cardiology

(AEPC), International Society for Heart and Lung Transplantation (ISHLT). *Eur Heart J.* 2016 Jan 1; 37(1):67-119.

Guerin, L., Couturaud, F., Parent, F., Revel, M. P., Gillaizeau, F., Planquette, B., Pontal, D., Guégan, M., Simonneau, G., Meyer, G. M., Sanches, O. Prevalence of chronic thromboembolic pulmonary hypertension after acute pulmonary embolism. Prevalence of CTEPH after pulmonary embolism. *Thromb. Haemost.* 2014, 112, 598–605.

Henkens, I. R., Mouchaers, K. T., Vonk-Noordegraaf, A., Boonstra, A., Swenne, C. A., Maan, A. C., Man, S. C., Twisk, J. W., van der Wall, E. E., Schalij, M. J., Vliegen, H. W. Improved ECG detection of presence and severity of right ventricular pressure load validated with cardiac magnetic resonance imaging. *Am J Physiol Heart Circ Physiol* 2008;294:H2150–H2157.

Hoeper, M. M., Mayer, E., Simonneau, G., Rubin, L. J. Chronic Thromboembolic Pulmonary hypertension. Contemporary Reviews in cardiovascular medicine; *Circulation* 2006:113:2011-2020.

Humbert, M., Simonneau, G., Pittrow, D., Delcroix, M., Pepke-Zaba, J., Langleben, D., Mielniczuk, L. M., Subias, P. E., Snijder, R. J., Barberà, J. A., Klotsche, J., Meier, C., Hoeper, M. M. Oral anticoagulants (NOAC and VKA) in chronicthromboembolic pulmonary hypertension. *J Heart Lung Transplant* 2022; 41: 716–721.

Humbert, M., Kovacs, G., Hoeper, M. M., Badagliacca, R., Berger, R. M., Brida, M., Carlsen, J., Coats, A. J., Escribano-Subias, P., Ferrari, P., Ferreira, D. S., Ghofrani, H. A., Giannakoulas, G., Kiely, D. G., Mayer, E., Meszaros, G., Nagavci, B., Olsson, K. M., epke-Zaba, J., Quint, J. K., Rådegran, G., Simonneau, G., Sitbon, O., Tonia, T., Toshner, M., Vachiery, J. L., Noordegraaf, A. V., Delcroix, M., Rosenkranz, M. ESC/ERS Scientific Document Group. 2022 ESC/ERS Guidelines for diagnosis and treatment of pulmonary hypertension; *Eur Respir J.* 2023 Jan 6;61(1):2200879.

Jones, N., Burns, A. T., Prior, D. L., Echocardiographic Assessment of the Right Ventricle–State of the Art; Heart, *Lung and Circulation* (2019) 28, 1339–1350.

Kawakami, T., Ogawa, A., Miyaji, K., Mizoguchi, H., Shimokawahara, H., Naito, T., Oka, T., Yunoki, K., Munemasa, M., Matsubara, H. Novel angiographic classification of each vascular lesion in chronic thromboembolic pulmonary hypertension based on selective angiogram and results of balloon pulmonary angioplasty. *Circ Cardiovasc Interv.* 2016;9(10):e003318.

Kim, E. Y., Seo, J. B., Assessment of Perfusion Pattern and Extent of Perfusion Defect on Dual-Energy CT Angiography: Correlations between the Causes of Pulmonary Hypertension and Vascular Parameters; *Korean J Radiol.* 2014 Mar-Apr;15(2):286-294.

Klok, F. A., Surie, S., Kempf, T., Eikenboom, J., van Straalen, J. P., van Kralingen, K. W., van Dijk, A. P., Vliegen, H. W., Bresser, P., Wollert, K. C., Huisman, M. V. A simple non-invasive diagnostic algorithm for ruling out chronic thromboembolic pulmonary hypertension in patients after acute pulmonary embolism. *Thromb Res* 2011;128:21–26.

Kovacs, G., Avian, A., Foris, V., Tscherner, M., Kqiku, X., Douschan, P., Bachmaier, G., Olschewski, A., Matucci-Cerinic, M., Olschewski, H. Use of ECG and other simple non-invasive tools to assess pulmonary hypertension. *PLoS One* 2016.

Konstantinides, S. V., Meyer, G., Becattini, C., Bueno, H., Geersing, G. J., Harjola, V. P., Huisman, M. V., Humbert, M., Jennings, C. S., Jiménez, D., Kucher, N., Lang, I. M., Lankeit, M., Lorusso, R., Mazzolai, L., Meneveau, N., Áinle, F. N., Prandoni, P., Pruszczyk, P., Righini, M., Torbicki, A., Belle, E. V., Zamorano, J. L., ESC Scientific Document Group. ESC Guidelines for the diagnosis and management of acute pulmonary embolism developed in collaboration with the European Respiratory Society (ERS). *Eur Heart J.* 2020 Jan 21;41(4):543-603.

Konstantinides, S. V., Torbicki, A., Agnelli, G., Danchin, N., Fitzmaurice, D., Galiè, N., Gibbs, J. S., Huisman, M. V., Humbert, M., Kucher, N., Lang, I., Lankeit, M., Lekakis, J., Maack, C., Meneveau, N., Perrier, A., Pruszczyk, P., Rasmussen, L. H., Schindler, T. H., Svitil, P., Noordegraaf, A. V., Zamorano, J. L., Zompatori, M. 2014 ESC Guidelines on the diagnosis and management of acute pulmonary embolism: The Task Force for the Diagnosis and Management of Acute Pulmonary Embolism of the European Society of Cardiology (ESC, Endorsed by the European Respiratory Society (ERS); *European Heart Journal*, (2014)35,3033–3080.

Kreitner, K. F., Ley, S., Kauczor, H. U., Mayer, E., Kramm, T., Pitton, M. B., Krummenauer, F., Thelen, M.: CTEPH: pre and postoperative assessment with breath-hold MR imaging techniques. Radiology 2004; 232(2):535-543.

Lang, I. M., Simonneau, G., Pepke-Zaba, J. W., Mayer, E., Ambroz, D., Blanco, I., Torbicki, A., Mellemkjaer, S., Yaici, A., Delcroix, M. Factors associated with diagnosis and operability of chronic thromboembolic pulmonary hypertension. A casecontrol study. *Thromb Haemost* 2013;110:83-91.

Lang, I. M., Campean, I. A., Sadushi-Kolici, R., Badr-Eslam, R., Gerges, C., Skoro-Sajer, N.. Chronic thromboembolic disease and chronic thromboembolic pulmonary hypertension; *Clin Chest Med* 42(2021) 81-90.

Lang, R. M., Badano, L. P., Mor-Avi, V., Afilalo, J., Armstrong, A., Ernande, L., Flachskampf, F. A., Foster, E., Goldstein, S. A., Kuznetsova, T., Lancellotti, P., Muraru, D., Picard, M. H., Rietzschel, E. R., Rudski. L., Spencer, K. T., Tsang, W., Voigt, J. U. Recommendations for Cardiac Chamber Quantification by Echocardiography in Adults: An Update from the American Society of Echocardiography and the European Association of Cardiovascular Imaging; *J Am Soc Echocardiogr*Volume 28 Number 1, 2015.

Leber, L., Beaudet, A., Muller, A. Epidemiology of pulmonary arterial hypertension and chronic thromboembolic pulmonary hypertension: identification of the most accurate estimates from a systematic literature review. *Pulm Circ* 2021; Jan 7;11(1): 2045894020977300.

Mahmud, E., Madani, M. M., Kim, N. H., Poch, D., Ang, L., Behnamfar, O., Patel, M. P., Auger, W. R. Chronic tromboembolic pulmonary hypertension; *JACC* vol. 71, No 21, 2018.

Miller. D, Makhoul, K., Foster, A. and Hosna AU. Chronic thromboembolic hypertension resulting in decompensated right heart failure: *J. Pulmonol Respir Res*. 2022;6:012-016.

Mizoguchi, H., Ogawa, A., Munemasa, M., Mikouchi, H., Ito, H., Matsubara, H. Refined Balloon Pulmonary Angioplasty for Inoperable Patients with Chronic

Thromboembolic Pulmonary Hypertension. *Circ. Cardiovasc. Interv.* 2012, 5, 748–755.

Morris, T. A., Fernandes, T. M., Channick, R.: How we do it: evaluation of dyspnea and exercise intolerance after acute pulmonary embolism. *Chest.* Open Access, July 2, 2022.

Nishiyama, K. H., Saboo, S. S., Tanabe, Y., Jasinowodolinski, D., Landay, M .J., Kay, F. U. Chronic pulmonary embolism:diagnosis. *Cardiovasc DiagnTher.* 2018;8(3):253-271.

Pepke-Zaba, J., Delcroix, M., Lang, I., Mayer, E., Jansa, P., Ambroz, D., Treacy, C., D'Armini, A. M., Morsolini, M., Snijder, R., Bresser, P., Torbicki, A., Kristensen, B., Lewczuk, J., Simkova, I., Barbera, J. A., de Perrot, M., Hoeper, M. M., Gaine, S., Speich, R., Gomez-Sanchez, M. A., Kovacs, G., Hamid, A. M., Jais, X., Simonneau, G. Chronic thromboembolic pulmonary hypertension (CTEPH): results from an international prospective registry. *Circulation*2011;124:1973-1981.

Pepke-Zaba, J., Hoeper, M. M., Humbert, M. Chronic thromboembolic pulmonary hypertension: Advances from bench to patient management. *Eur. Respir. J.* 2013, 41, 8–9.

Poor, H., Serrao, G., Grapsa, J., Chandrashekhar, Y. S., Bianco, A., Lookstein, R. A., Fuster, V. High risk pulmonary embolism during labor; *JACC Case* reports; (2023) Vol. 6: 1-9.

Quarck, R., Wynants, M., Verbeken, E., Meyns, B., Delcroix, M. Contribution of inflammation and impaired angiogenesis to the pathobiology of chronic thromboembolic pulmonary hypertension. *Eur. Respir. J.* 2015, 46, 431–443.

Ruaro, B., Baratella, E. Chronic Thromboembolic Pulmonary Hypertension: An Update; *Diagnostics* 2022, 12, 235.

Ruaro, B., Confalonieri, P., Caforio, G., Baratella, E., Pozzan, R., Tavano, S., Bozzi, C., Lerda, S., Geri, P., Biolo, M., Cortale, M., Confalonieri, M., Salton, F. Chronic Thromboembolic Pulmonary Hypertension: an observationalstudy; *Medicina* 2022, 58, 1094.

Rudski, L. G., Lai, W. W, Afilalo, J., Hua, L, Handschumacher, M. D., Chandrasekaran, K., Solomon, S. D., Louie, E. L, Schiller, N. B., Guidelines for the Echocardiographic Assessment of the Right Heart in Adults: A Report from the American Society of Echocardiography Endorsed by the European Association of Echocardiography, a registered branch of the European Society of Cardiology, and the Canadian Society of Echocardiography; *J Am Soc Echocardiogr* 2010; 23:685-713.

Simonneau, G., D'Armini, A. M., Grimminger, F., Hoeper, M. M., Jansa, P., Kim, N. H., Wang, C., Wilkins, M. R., Fritsch, A., Davie, N., Colorado, P., Mayer, E. Riociguat for treatment of chronic thromboembolic pulmonary hypertension: a long-term extension study (CHEST 2). *Eur Resp J.* 2015; 45:1293-1302.

Simonneau, G., Dorfmüller, R., Guignabert, C., Mercier, O., and Humbert, M. Chronic thromboembolic pulmonary hypertension: the magic of pathophysiology; *Annals of cardiothoracic surgery*, Vol. 11, No 2, 2022.

Simonneau, G., Fadel, E., Noordegraaf, A. V., Toshner, M., Lang, I. M., Klok, F. A., McInnis, M. C., Screaton, N., Madani, M. M., Martinez, G., Salaunkey, K., Jenkins, D. P., Matsubara, H., Brénot, P., Hoeper, M. M., Ghofrani, H. A., Jaïs, X., Wiedenroth,

C. B., Guth, S., Kim, N. H., Pepke-Zaba, J., Delcroix, J. M., Mayer, E. Highlights from the International chronic thromboembolic pulmonary hypertension congress 2021; *Eur Respir Rev* 2023;32:220132.

Srbinovska Kostovska, E. Role of echocardiography in diagnosis of pulmonary hypertension; *Cardiol Croat.* 2013;8(7-8):258-263.

Swietlik, E. M., Ruggiero, A., Fletcher, A. J., Taboada, D., Knightbridge, E., Harlow, L., Harvey, I., Screaton, N., Cannon, J. E., Sheares, K. K. K., Choo, N. G., Jenkins, Pepke-Zaba, D. P., Toshner, M. R. Limitations of resting haemodynamics in chronic thromboembolic disease without pulmonary hypertension. *Eur Respir J* 2019; 53: 1801787.

Chapter 10

Cancer-Associated Venous Thromboembolism

Sonja Salinger*, **PhD**
Cardiology Clinic, Clinical Center Nis, Serbia

Abstract

Cancer-associated venous thromboembolism (VTE) represents one of the major causes of increased morbidity and mortality in cancer patients. Although significant advances have been made in the treatment of VTE, optimal medical therapy in cancer patients still remains a major challenge to clinicians due to the high incidence of symptomatic and asymptomatic pulmonary embolism (PE), increased recurrence episodes, worsened predicted survival, increased hemorrhage risk, and several drug interactions. It is very important to determine the risk level in order to adequately treat the patients, but also select the patients for primary and secondary prevention of VTE and assess the risk of early death in case of acute pulmonary embolism. Nowadays, the significant development in VTE treatment in cancer patients is evident. Direct oral anticoagulants (DOACs) simplified the treatment of VTE compared to low-molecular-weight heparin (LMWH) due to their characteristics, way of administration, fixed-dose regimens and lower cost. However, their prescription requires additional caution, especially in patients with gastrointestinal malignancies. The latest available data on reperfusion therapy emphasize the importance of an individual approach to each cancer patient with VTE. The aim of this chapter is to present recent insight into VTE treatment, risk stratification for thromboprophylaxis and clinical approach in patients with cancer and suspected or established VTE.

* Corresponding Author's Email: sonja.salinger@gmail.com.

In: Pulmonary Embolism
Editors: Irena Mitevska, Sonja Salinger, Marijan Bosevski et al.
ISBN: 979-8-89113-175-0

Keywords: cancer, pulmonary thromboembolism, risk stratification, therapy

Introduction

Cancer-associated venous thromboembolism (VTE), which includes deep vein thrombosis, pulmonary embolism, and central venous catheter-related VTE, is the second leading cause of death in patients with cancer after progression. The prevalence of cancer-associated thrombosis is increasing due to numerous factors, including prolonged patient survival, anticancer therapies, enhanced detection of incidental VTE during surveillance imaging, and broader use of central venous catheters (Farge et al., 2022).

The risk of developing VTE in cancer patients is increased up to sevenfold compared to the general population (Nahla et al., 2018). Symptomatic acute VTE is a common complication in cancer patients. It occurs in up to 15% of cancer patients during their disease course. However, VTEs are incidentally detected in about one-half of all cancer patients without any clinical suspicion of VTE at the time of diagnosis (Van der Hulle et al., 2014). Patients with cancer-associated thrombosis are at high risk of recurrent VTE and anticoagulant-related bleeding, associated with high morbidity and resource use (Farge et al., 2022).

The occurrence of VTE in patients with cancer may interfere with planned chemotherapy regimens, increase the risk of mortality, and result in increased costs compared with patients without cancer (Lyman et al., 2021). However, the impact of VTE extends beyond the physical and economic; it also significantly affects cancer patients' quality of life, leading to considerable distress to patients with cancer and their families. More than 50% of thrombotic events occur within 3 months of the cancer diagnosis, by the time when most cancer treatments are underway. Patients, who are still coming to terms with a recent cancer diagnosis, often view the occurrence of VTE as a further threat to life, confirmation of the severity of their condition, and a poor prognostic sign (Lyman et al., 2021, Font et al., 2018).

Risk Factors for VTE

VTE risk factors in cancer patients can be grouped into 3 general categories: intrinsic and extrinsic patient-related factors, cancer-related factors, and treatment-related factors (Nahla AM et al., 2018). The risk for VTE and recurrent VTE is highest among certain hematologic malignancies, such as lymphoma, acute leukemia, and multiple myeloma. Patients with high-grade lymphoma and acute promyelocytic leukemia appear to be at higher risk than other forms of lymphoma or leukemia. Lung cancer, gastrointestinal cancer (stomach/colon), pancreatic cancer, kidney cancer, bone cancer, myelodysplastic disorder, and patients with distant metastasis are also susceptible (NCCN Guidelines, 2021). However, cancers originating at the sites, such as head, neck, and bladder, had no high prevalence of associated VTE (Nahla al., 2018, NCCN Guidelines, 2021, Stein et al., 2016).

Several risk factors for developing venous thrombosis usually coexist in cancer patients, including surgery, hospital admissions, immobilization, and the presence of the central catheter, older age, platelet count $\geq 350x10^9/L$, hemoglobin<100 g/L or use of red cell growth factors, and leukocyte count $\geq$ 11 X 10^9 /L 35 kg/m^2 (Nahla et al., 2018, Khorana et al., 2007). A review of cancer patients who underwent surgery showed that they had twice the risk of postoperative deep venous thrombosis (DVT) as non-cancer patients who underwent similar procedures. Risk factors may be closely connected. The risk of VTE increases with age and is also associated with malignancy. Among cancer patients undergoing surgery, advanced age, disability, prolonged and difficult surgery, and a lengthy and complicated postoperative course add to the risk of DVT (Nahla et al., 2018, NCCN Guidelines, 2021, Khorana et al., 2007).

The extent of cancer impacts the risk of VTE. Chemotherapy and radiation increase the risk of VTE (Lyman et al., 2021; Agnelli et al., 2006). Chemotherapy such as thalidomide/lenalidomide/pomalidomide in combination with high-dose dexamethasone (480 mg/ month) or doxorubicin or multiagent chemotherapy in myeloma patients, exogenous hormonal therapies such as tamoxifen/raloxifene, dicthylstilbestrol and new molecular targeted therapies are well-established risk factors for venous thromboembolism. The risk of VTE in cancer patients is increased by concomitant risk factors such as factor V Leiden mutation or prothrombin 20210A mutation, as well as by the presence of other comorbid features that influence the overall thrombotic complications in non-cancerous patients (Nahlaet al., 2018, Ha et al., 2017).

Besides antineoplastic therapies, certain supportive care measures used in cancer treatment may also increase the risk of VTE, including red blood cell transfusions, as well as erythropoietin-stimulating agents for managing anemia for patients undergoing cancer treatment (Bohlius at al., 2006).

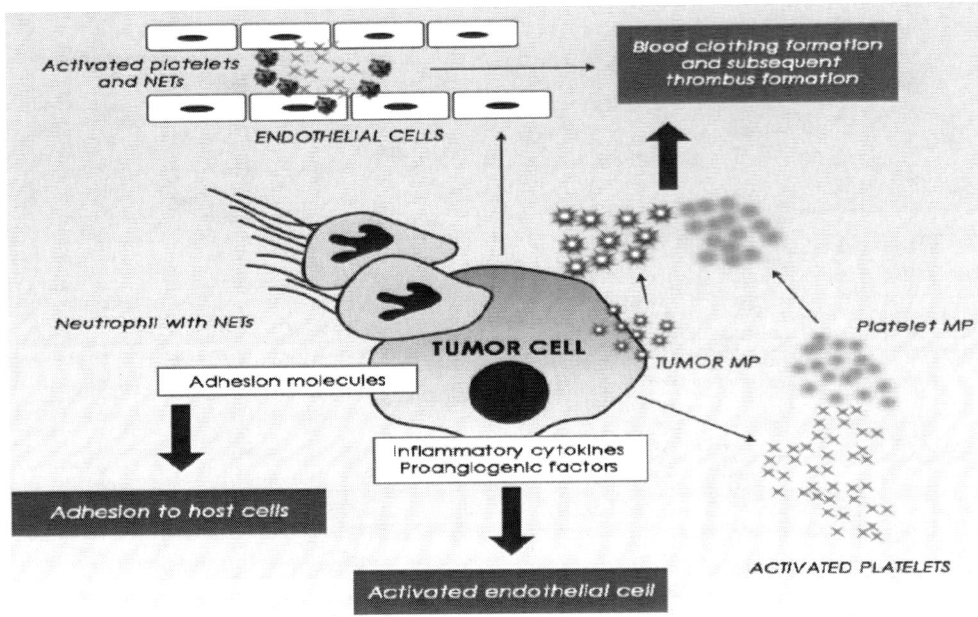

Figure 1. Cancer-hemostatic system interrelation. Tumor cells may stimulate the hemostatic system in numerous ways. Tumor cells release procoagulant activities, and microparticles (MP), by which the coagulation cascade is activated. Tumor cells also activate the host hemostatic cells (endothelial cells, leukocytes, and thrombocytes) either by releasing soluble factors or by direct adherence. In this way, the expression of a procoagulant phenotype of these cells is evoked. Besides, neutrophils may release neutrophil extracellular traps (NETs), and the adherence of a great number of NETs to the vasculature may trigger thrombosis by providing a platform for platelet adhesion, activation, and thrombin generation. Reproduced with permission from (12) Bisceglia, 2017.

Pathophysiological Mechanism of Cancer-Induced Thromboembolism

Several mechanisms may be involved in the pathogenesis of thromboembolic events in patients with cancer. These include (1) tumor cell procoagulants or cytokines, (2) tumor-associated inflammatory cell procoagulants and/or cytokines, and (3) mediators of platelet adhesion or aggregation generated by tumor cells or tumor-associated inflammatory cells. Stasis and endothelial damage may also be involved in the pathogenesis of thromboembolic events in patients with cancer (Bisceglia et al., 2017).

Cancer cells and the coagulation system are interrelated. General prothrombotic mechanisms are related both to the host response to cancer and the procoagulant activity of cancer cells (Figure 1). Host-related factors include the acute-phase reaction, paraprotein production, inflammation, necrosis, and hemodynamic disorders. Malignant cells can activate blood coagulation in several ways. They can produce procoagulant factors such as tissue factor (TF) and cancer procoagulant factor (CP), which are the most powerful procoagulant observed; microparticles (MP); inflammatory cytokines such as tumor necrosis factor (TNF) and interleukin-1 (IL-1); pro-angiogenic factors as vascular endothelial growth factor (VEGF), which promotes both endothelial prothrombotic alterations and angiogenesis. VEGF is an indirect procoagulant that increases microvascular permeability, reprograms gene expression, and promotes the survival of endothelial cells; the resulting increased vascular density plays a key role in the pathophysiology of many cancers. The same procoagulant factors contribute to tumor progression. Also, platelets, endothelial cells, and neutrophils of host cells are stimulated to express procoagulant activity. Thus, thromboembolism frequently worsens the course of malignancy and may be the first symptom of cancer (Bisceglia et al., 2017, Falanga et al., 2015).

The identification of multiple factors, including biomarkers, associated with the risk of cancer-associated VTE has prompted the development of risk scores for predicting VTE and its complications (Khorana et al., 2008).

Assessment of the Thrombotic Risk in Cancer Patients

The Khorana score is based on five predictive models, including cancer sites, platelet counts, hemoglobin level or the use of erythropoiesis-stimulating agents, leukocyte count, and body mass index (Khorana et al., 2008). Risk predictor models involve the Ottawa score, which identifies patients at the highest risk of recurrent VTE and who may benefit from prolonged anticoagulation treatment among those with cancer- associated VTE, and the Khorana score for chemotherapy-associated VTE (Delluc et al., 2020).

Anticoagulation Therapy

Patients with cancer frequently have both an increased thrombotic risk and an increased hemorrhage risk associated with certain cancer locations (e.g., gastrointestinal (GI), intracranial), thrombocytopenia, and other coagulation defects (secondary to bone marrow invasion, cancer therapies, or cancer itself) and associated comorbidities (e.g., renal or hepatic dysfunction, GI toxicities). Several anticancer agents are further characterized by drug interactions with anticoagulants. Thromboembolic risk, hemorrhage risk, drug interactions and patient preferences (TBIP acronym) may render anticoagulation in cancer in a quite challenging way (Lyon et al., 2022). The initial treatment approach for VTE in cancer patients is shown in Table 1. The approach to early and long-term treatment of VTE in cancer patients is shown in Table 2.

Since 2019 when ITAC guidelines were published, three randomized clinical trials and 12 meta-analyses have assessed the efficacy and safety of LMWHs or direct oral anticoagulants for the treatment of cancer-associated thrombosis (Farge et al., 2022, Farge et al., 2019). The initial treatment of established VTE (up to 10 days) included LMWHs, unfractionated heparin, or fondaparinux (followed by a vitamin K antagonist). An increased number of patients with cancer-associated thrombosis receiving LMWHs (n=1840) in six randomized clinical trials comparing direct oral anticoagulants with LMWH resulted in an upgrade from 1B to 1A for LMWHs as an initial treatment in the first 5–10 days (Yan et al., 2020). Direct oral anticoagulants rivaroxaban or edoxaban were recommended (grade 1B) in 2019 as the initial treatment options in patients with cancer-associated thrombosis who were not at high risk of gastrointestinal or genitourinary bleeding. Fondaparinux and unfractionated heparin remain acceptable alternative treatment options without new evidence.

Table 1. Initial treatment of established VTE (up to 10 days of anticoagulation) in cancer patients

LMWH once daily (eGFR ≥ 30 mL/min) (grade 1A). Enoxaparin (1 mg/kg), twice-daily in high risk of bleeding, moderate renal failure, the need for technical intervention surgery or changing regimen.
Rivaroxaban or apixaban (in the first 10 days), or edoxaban (started after at least 5 days of parenteral anticoagulation) for patients who do not have a high risk of gastrointestinal or genitourinary bleeding (eGFR ≥ 30 mL/min). (grade 1A)
UFH when LMWH or direct oral anticoagulants are contraindicated/not available (grade 2C)
Fondaparinux (grade 2D)
Thrombolysis can only be considered on a case-by-case basis (contraindications – brain metastasis)
Inferior vena cava filters when anticoagulant treatment is contraindicated or, in the case of pulmonary embolism, when recurrence occurs under optimal anticoagulation.

Abbreviations: LMWH- low molecular weight heparin; GFR- glomerular filtration rate; UFH-unfractionated heparin.

Table 2. Early (up to 6 months) and long-term (beyond 6 months) maintenance

LMWHs are preferred over vitamin K antagonists
Direct oral anticoagulants (edoxaban, rivaroxaban, or apixaban) in the absence of strong drug interactions or gastrointestinal absorption impairment (eGFR ≥30 mL/min) (grade 1A). Caution in patients with gastrointestinal tract malignancies, especially upper gastrointestinal tract malignancies,
LMWH or direct oral anticoagulants should be used for a minimum of 6 months (grade 1A).
Termination or continuation of anticoagulation should be based on individual evaluation of the benefit–risk ratio, tolerability, drug availability, patient preference, and cancer activity.

Abbreviations: LMWH- low molecular weight heparin; GFR- glomerular filtration rate.

Table 3. Prophylaxis of VTE in surgically-treated patients with cancer

LMWH once daily (eGFR ≥ 30 mL/min) (grade 1A).
Low-dose UFH three times per day
There is insufficient evidence to support fondaparinux (grade 2C) or direct oral anticoagulants (grade 2B) as an alternative to LMWH for the prophylaxis of postoperative VTE in patients with cancer.
Highest prophylactic dose of LMWH to prevent postoperative VTE
Extended prophylaxis (4 weeks) with LMWH after major abdominal or pelvic surgery (either laparotomy or laparoscopy) who do not have a high risk of bleeding (grade 1A)
Mechanical methods are not recommended as monotherapy except when pharmacological methods are contraindicated (grade 2A).
Inferior vena cava filters are not recommended for routine prophylaxis (grade 1A).

Abbreviations: LMWH- low molecular weight heparin; GFR- glomerular filtration rate; VTE- venous trhomboembolism.

Table 4. Prophylaxis of VTE in medically-treated patients with cancer

LMWH or fondaparinux if eGFR ≥ 30 mL/min or UFH
LMWH (grade 1A) or DOAC (rivaroxaban or apixaban; grade 1B) in ambulatory patients with locally advanced or metastatic pancreatic cancer treated with systemic anticancer therapy and low risk of bleeding.
LMWH is not recommended for patients with locally advanced or metastatic lung cancer treated with systemic anticancer therapy, and low risk of bleeding
DOAC (rivaroxaban or apixaban) in ambulatory patients who are receiving systemic anticancer therapy and are at intermediate to high risk of VTE (Khorana score ≥ 2), and not actively bleeding or not high risk for bleeding (grade 1B).
In patients with myeloma treated with immunomodulatory drugs combined with steroids or other systemic anticancer therapies, VTE primary pharmacological prophylaxis is recommended (grade 1A); vitamin K antagonists at low or therapeutic doses and apixaban at prophylactic doses), LMWH at prophylactic doses, or low-dose aspirin (100 mg daily) (grade 2B).

Abbreviations: LMWH- low molecular weight heparin; UFH-unfractionated heparin; DOAC- direct oral anticoagulant VTE-venous thromboembolism.

Primary Prevention of Venous Thromboembolism

Patients undergoing surgery and those hospitalized or on prolonged bed rest require thromboprophylaxis with low-dose anticoagulation therapy (Xin et al., 2020). The ENOXACAN (Enoxaparin and Cancer) II study showed favorable outcomes with LMWH as primary thromboprophylaxis for 4 weeks after major abdominal or pelvic cancer surgery. In ambulatory patients, VTE risk should be individually determined, and the proposed scores, such as the Khorana or the COMPASS-CAT (prospective Comparison of Methods for thromboembolic risk assessment with clinical Perceptions and Awareness in real-life patients Cancer Associated Thrombosis) score, may be useful (Gerotziafas et al., 2017). Further trials and a meta-analysis have shown that LMWH significantly reduced the incidence of symptomatic VTE in ambulatory patients with cancer receiving chemotherapy with satisfactory safety. Prophylaxis of VTE in surgically and medically treated cancer patients is shown in Tables 3 and 4.

Two randomized, placebo-controlled, double-blind clinical trials have assessed the role of DOAC in the primary prevention of VTE in high-risk ambulatory patients receiving systemic cancer therapy (Khorana score ≥ 2). Over a follow-up period of 180 days, apixaban (2.5 mg twice a day) therapy resulted in a significantly lower rate of VTE, although the rate of major bleeding episodes was higher than with a placebo. Rivaroxaban (10 mg once a day) treatment resulted in a non-significantly lower incidence of VTE or death due to VTE with low hemorrhage risk (no significant differences with a placebo). Further data on the use of DOAC in this setting are warranted. Patients should be thoroughly informed about the advantages and disadvantages of such a therapy, cancer prognosis, drug cost, and duration of prophylaxis (Lyon et al., 2022). Treatment of recurrent PE episodes and prophylaxis of cathcter base thrombosis in cancer patients is shown in Tables 5 and 6.

Table 5. Treatment of VTE recurrence in patients with cancer under anticoagulation

Increase LMWH by 20–25% or switch to direct oral anticoagulants
For direct oral anticoagulants, switch to LMWH
For vitamin K antagonist, switch to LMWH or direct oral anticoagulants

Abbreviations: LMWH- low molecular weight heparin.

Table 6. Prophylaxis of catheter-related thrombosis

Use of anticoagulation for routine prophylaxis of catheter-related thrombosis is not recommended (grade 1A).
Catheters should be inserted on the right side, in the jugular vein, and the distal extremity of the central catheter should be located at the junction of the superior vena cava and the right atrium (grade 1B).
In patients requiring central venous catheters, the use of implanted ports is suggested.

Treatment and Secondary Prevention of Venous Thromboembolism

Several large RCTs and meta-analyses have shown that LMWH decreases the risk of recurrent VTE by 40% compared to VKA, with a similar risk of major hemorrhage. However, VKAs are characterized by an unpredictable anticoagulation effect and low time in therapeutic range in patients with malignancies due to multiple drug interactions, GI toxicity, malnutrition, and liver dysfunction. DOAC have been assessed as potential alternatives to LMWH for cancer-associated VTE, based on RCTs that compared edoxaban, rivaroxaban, or apixaban to dalteparin (Lyon et al., 2022). The totality of evidence from four randomized clinical trials (ADAM-VTE, CARAVAGGIO, CASTA-DIVA, and CANVAS) found that direct oral anticoagulants are non-inferior to LMWHs for the outcomes of recurrent VTE and mortality (Farge et al., 2022, Lyon, 2022). The risk of major bleeding was similar, although DOACs were associated with an increased risk of clinically relevant non-major bleeding, particularly in patients with luminal GI and genitourinary malignancies (Sabatino et al., 2020). As a result, edoxaban, rivaroxaban, and apixaban are recommended for the treatment of VTE (DVT and PE) in patients with cancer without any of the following bleeding risk factors: unoperated GI or GU malignancies, history of recent bleeding or within 7 days of major surgery, significant thrombocytopenia (platelet count, 50 000/μL), severe renal dysfunction (creatinine clearance (CrCl, 15 mL/min), or GI comorbidities. In addition, drug interactions between DOAC, cancer therapies, and other concomitant treatments should be checked (Lyon et al., 2022). There are also concerns about DOAC in patients with GI toxicity, such as vomiting or those having undergone gastrectomy or extensive intestine resection, as well as those with severely impaired renal function. Shared decision-making considering informed patient preferences should guide the choice of anticoagulation. Incidentally encountered proximal DVT or PE should be treated in the same manner as symptomatic VTE, as they bear similar rates of recurrence and mortality (Den et al., 2011). The minimal duration of anticoagulation is 6 months, and extended anticoagulation is suggested in the presence of active malignancy, metastatic disease, or chemotherapy use. Cohort studies have shown that extended LMWH therapy beyond 6 and up to 12 months is safe in cancer-associated VTE (Lyon et al., 2022, Francis et al., 2015). However, patients with cancer are also at high risk of hemorrhage during anticoagulant treatment and a periodic assessment of the risk/benefit ratio should be performed. In VTE relapse under anticoagulation, the patient should be investigated for treatment adherence, cancer progression, or relapse, while a different anticoagulation strategy should be endorsed (e.g., replacement of DOAC with LMWH) The management of patients with VTE and a platelet count < 25 000/µL should be individualized (Key et al., 2020). The duration of anticoagulation in patients with catheter-associated thrombosis depends upon whether the catheter is removed or remains in situ. If removed, then anticoagulation should continue for a minimum of 3 months, and until follow-up cardiac imaging confirms the resolution of the thrombus. If the catheter remains in situ, then long-term therapeutic anticoagulation should continue.

Inferior Vena Cava Filters

The recommendation from ITAC guidelines for inferior vena cava filters has been unchanged since 2019 (Farge et al., 2022, Font C et al., 2018). A new retrospective database study, which used propensity score matching and competing risk analysis, compared 33,740 patients with cancer and concomitant deep vein thrombosis who had inferior vena cava filters with 54 845 patients without inferior vena cava filters, showing improved pulmonary embolism-free survival (hazard ratio [HR] 0·69, 95% CI 0·64–0·75; $p < 0{\cdot}001$), without increased risk of recurrent deep vein thrombosis (Angelini et al., 2019). Another propensity-matched retrospective study compared the use of inferior vena cava filters in 247 patients with cancer in whom anticoagulant therapy was contraindicated, with 247 matched patients with cancer but without inferior vena cava filters, reporting a non-significant lower risk of death (12·2% vs. 17·0%, $p = 0{\cdot}13$), and a significantly lower risk of pulmonary embolism-related mortality (0·8% vs. 4·0%; $p = 0{\cdot}04$), (Quezada et al., 2020).

Bleeding Complications

Bleeding complications are more common in patients with cancer than in patients without cancer. This may be directly related to the tumor itself, or indirectly related to chemotherapy- or RT-induced weakening of mucosal barriers (Steffelet al., 2021). GI and genitourinary cancers in high-risk patients are associated with a significant excess bleeding risk compared with other solid tumors (Angelini D et al., 2019). Thrombocytopenia and platelet dysfunction due to hematological malignancies or bone marrow suppression may deteriorate bleeding. Other bleeding risk factors include advancing age, renal or hepatic impairment, metastatic disease, low body mass index, and treatment with ibrutinib, VEGFi, cetuximab, or bevacizumab (Steffel et al., 2021, Angelini et al., 2019). Gastric protection with routine proton pump inhibitor use should be considered in all patients with cancer on DAPT or anticoagulation (Steffel et al., 2021, Roule et al., 2020). Treatment of catheter-related VTE and VTE in unique situations are shown in Tables 7 and 8.

Table 7. Treatment of established catheter-related thrombosis

LMWHs for a minimum of 3 months and as long as the central venous catheter is in place
In patients with cancer and with catheter-related thrombosis, the central venous catheter can be kept in place if it is functional, well-positioned, and not infected

Abbreviations: LMWH- low molecular weight heparin.

Management of Bleeding

Basic principles of bleeding management should be followed with control of the bleeding source whenever possible. Platelet transfusions for significant thrombocytopenia and withholding and reversal of anticoagulation for life-threatening bleeding may be needed as in the general population (Steffel et al., 2021). Antifibrinolytic agents, such as tranexamic acid or e-aminocaproic acid, can be considered. Non-specific support of hemostasis using coagulation factor concentrates and specific reversal agents may be needed for patients treated with DOAC and life-threatening bleeding. Recombinant activated factor VII or activated prothrombin complex concentrates should be avoided in patients with recent thrombosis.

Table 8. Treatment of venous thromboembolism (VTE) in unique situations

In patients with a brain tumor, LMWH or DOAC can be used for the treatment (grade 2A).
LMWH or UFH postoperatively for the prevention of VTE in patients with cancer undergoing neurosurgery
Primary pharmacological prophylaxis of VTE in medically treated patients with a brain tumor who are not undergoing neurosurgery is not recommended (grade 1B).
If eGFR < 30 mL/min, UFH followed by early VKA (possible from day 1) or LMWH adjusted to anti-Xa concentration for the treatment of established VTE
If eGFR < 30 mL/min, an external compression device can be applied, pharmacological prophylaxis could be considered on a case-by-case basis; UFH can be used on a case-by-case basis
Full doses of anticoagulant can be used for the treatment of established VTE if the platelet count is > 50×10^9 per L and there is no evidence of bleeding; for patients with a platelet count < 50×10^9 per L, decisions on treatment and dose should be made on a case-by-case basis with the utmost caution
If platelet count > 80×10^9 per L, pharmacological prophylaxis could be used; if the platelet count is < 80×10^9 per L, pharmacological prophylaxis can only be considered on a case-by-case basis and careful monitoring is recommended
In the CASSINI64 and AVERT65 trials, patients with a platelet count as low as 50×10^9 per L were allowed to receive thromboprophylaxis
In patients with cancer who are pregnant, LMWH for treatment of established VTE and for VTE prophylaxis is suggested; avoidance of vitamin K antagonists and direct oral anticoagulants
In obese patients, consideration for a higher dose of LMWH should be given for cancer surgery
For the treatment of symptomatic catheter-related thrombosis in children with cancer, anticoagulant treatment is recommended for a minimum of 3 months and as long as the central venous catheter is in place
In children with acute lymphoblastic leukemia undergoing induction chemotherapy, we recommend LMWH as thromboprophylaxis
In children requiring central venous catheters, we suggest the use of implanted ports over peripherally inserted central catheter lines

Abbreviations: LMWH- low molecular weight heparin; UFH-unfractionated heparin; DOAC- direct oral anticoagulant VTE-venous thromboembolism.

Recently published 2022 ITAC guidelines, endorsed by the International Society on Thrombosis and Hemostasis, and the new evidence on the treatment and prophylaxis of cancer-associated thrombosis, including in patients with cancer and with COVID-19 (Farge et al., 2022) are summarized in this chapter.

Conclusion

Cancer-associated venous thromboembolism (VTE), as one of the major causes of increased morbidity and mortality in cancer patients, represents great challenge to clinicians for treatment. Although significant advances have been made in the treatment of VTE, optimal medical therapy in cancer patients still remains a major challenge to clinicians. Presentation, recurrence, and bleeding risk emphasize many obstacles to achieving good balance between thrombotic and bleeding risk. Low-molecular-weight heparins is still the drug of choice for prevention and treatment of cancer-associated thrombosis. Novel anticoagulants as an effective alternative are highly recommended in therapeutic regimens. Optimal treatment requires a patient-based approach and precise insight into the risk/benefit ratio and drug interactions.

References

Agnelli, G., Bolis, G., Capussotti, L., Scarpa, R. M., Tonelli, F., Bonizzoni, E., Moia, M., Parazzini F., Rossi, R., Sonaglia, F., Valarani, B., Bianchini, C., Gussoni, G. A clinical outcome-based prospective study on venous thromboembolism after cancer surgery: the @RISTOS project. *Ann. Surg.* 2006; 243:89–95.

Angelini, D. E., Radivoyevitch, T., McCrae, K. R., Khorana, A. A. Bleeding incidence and risk factors among cancer patients treated with anticoagulation. *Am. J. Hematol.* 2019;94: 780–785.

Bisceglia, I., Maurea, N. *Thromboembolic Disorders as a Consequence of Cancer*. In. Lestuzzi C, Oliva S, Ferraù F, eds. Manual of Cardio-oncology. Springer International Publishing Switzerland 2017: Chapter 4:68-85.

Bohlius, J., Wilson, J., Seidenfeld, J., Piper, M., Schwarzer, G., Sandercock, J., Trelle, S., Weingart, O., Sue Bayliss, S., Djulbegovic, B., Bennett, C. L., Langensiepen, S., Hyde, C., Engert, A. Recombinant human erythropoietin's and cancer patients: updated meta-analysis of 57 studies including 9353 patients. *J. Natl. Cancer Inst.* 2006;98(10):708-714.

Delluc, A., Miranda, S., den Exter, P., Louzada, M., Alatri A., Ahn S, Monreal, M., Khorana, A., Huisman, M. V., Wells, P. S., Carrier, M. Accuracy of the Ottawa score in risk stratification of recurrent venous thromboembolism in patients with cancer-associated venous thromboembolism: a systematic review and meta-analysis. *Haematologica* 2020; 105(5):1436-1442.

Den Exter, P. L., Hooijer, J., Dekkers, O. M., Huisman, M. V. Risk of recurrent venous thromboembolism and mortality in patients with cancer incidentally diagnosed with pulmonary embolism: a comparison with symptomatic patients. *J. Clin. Oncol.* 2011; 29:2405–2409.

Falanga, A., Marchetti, M., Russo, L. The mechanisms of cancer-associated thrombosis. *Thromb. Res.* 2015;135 Suppl 1: S8–11.

Farge, D., Frere, C., Connors, J. M., Khorana, A. A., Kakkar, A., Ay, C., Muñoz, A., Brenner, B., Prata, P. H., Brilhante, D., Antic, D., Casais, P., Esposito, M. S. G., Ikezoe, T., Abutalib, S. A., Meillon-García, L., Bounameaux, H., Pabinger, I., Douketis, J., the International Initiative on Thrombosis and Cancer (ITAC) advisory panel. The International Initiative on Thrombosis and Cancer (ITAC) advisory panel. 2022 international clinical practice guidelines for the treatment and prophylaxis of venous thromboembolism in patients with cancer, including patients with COVID-19. *Lancet Oncol.* 2022 Jul;23(7): e334-e347.

Farge, D., Frere, C., Connors, J. M., Ay, C., Khorana, A. A., Munoz, A., Brenner, B., Kakkar, A., Rafii, H., Solymoss, S., Brilhante, D., Monreal, M., Bounameaux, H., Pabinger, I., Douketis, J. International Initiative on Thrombosis and Cancer (ITAC) advisory panel. 2019 international clinical practice guidelines for the treatment and prophylaxis of venous thromboembolism in patients with cancer. *Lancet Oncol.* 2019; 20: e566–e581.

Francis, C. W., Kessler, C. M., Goldhaber, S. Z., Kovacs, M. J., Monreal, M., Huisman, M. V., Bergqvist, D., Turpie, A. G., Ortel, T. L., Spyropoulos, A. C., Pabinger, I., Kakkar, A. K. Treatment of venous thromboembolism in cancer patients with dalteparin for up to 12 months: the DALTECAN Study. *J. Thromb. Haemost.* 2015; 13:1028–1035.

Font, C., Nelson, A., Garcia-Fernandez, T., Prout, H., Gee, P., Noble, S. Patients' experience of living with cancer-associated thrombosis in Spain (PELICANOS). *Support Care Cancer.* 2018;26(9):3233-3239.

Gerotziafas, G. T., Taher, A., Abdel-Razeq, H., AboElnazar, E., Spyropoulos, A. C., Shemmari, S. E., Larsen, A. K., Elalamy, I.; COMPASS–CAT Working Group et al. A predictive score for thrombosis associated with breast, colorectal, lung, or ovarian cancer: the prospective COMPASS–cancer associated thrombosis study. *Oncologist* 2017; 22:1222–1231.

Ha, N., Barnes, G. D. (2017). Optimal treatment approaches of cancer induced thrombosis, USA.

Lyman, G. H., Carrier, M., Ay, C., Di Nisio, M., Hicks, L. K., Khorana, A. A., Leavitt, A. D., Lee, A. Y. Y., Macbeth, F., Morgan, R. L., Noble, S., Sexton, E. A., Stenehjem, D., Wiercioch, W., Kahale, L. A., Alonso-Coello, P. American Society of Hematology 2021 guidelines for management of venous thromboembolism: prevention and treatment in patients with cancer. The American Society of Hematology 2021. *Blood Adv.* 2021;5(4):927-974.

Lyon, A., López-Fernández, T., Couch, L, Asteggiano, R., Aznar, M., Bergler-Klein, J., Boriani, G., Cardinale, D., Cordoba, R., Cosyns, B., Cutter, D., de Azambuja, E., de

Boer, R., Dent, S., Farmakis, D., Gevaert, S., Gorog, D., Herrmann, J., Lenihan, D., Moslehi, J., Moura, B., Salinger, S., Stephens, R., Suter, T., Szmit, S., Tamargo, J., Thavendiranathan, P., Tocchetti, C., van der, Meer, P., van der Pal, H.; ESC Scientific Document Group. 2022 ESC Guidelines on cardio-oncology developed in collaboration with the European Hematology Association (EHA), the European Society for Therapeutic Radiology and Oncology (ESTRO) and the International Cardio-Oncology Society (IC-OS) Developed by the task force on cardio-oncology of the European Society of Cardiology (ESC). *European Heart Journal* (2022) 00, 1–133 https://doi.org/10.1093/eurheartj/ehac244.

Key, N. S., Khorana, A. A., Kuderer, N. M., Bohlke, K., Lee, A. Y. Y., Arcelus, J. I., Wong, S. L., Balaban, E. P., Flowers, C. R., Francis, C. W., Gates, L. E., Kakkar, A. K., Levine, M. N., Liebman, H. A., Tempero, M. A., Lyman, G. H., Falanga, A. Venous thromboembolism prophylaxis and treatment in patients with cancer: ASCO clinical practice guideline update. *J. Clin. Oncol.* 2020;38: 496–520.

Khorana, A. A., Francis, C. W., Culakova, E., Kuderer, N. M., Lyman, G. H. Thromboembolism is a leading cause of death in cancer patients receiving outpatient chemotherapy. *J. Thromb. Haemost.* 2007;5: 632–634.

Khorana, A. A., Kuderer, N. M., Culakova, E., Lyman, G. H., Francis, C. W. Development and validation of a predictive model for chemotherapy-associated thrombosis. *Blood.* 2008;111(10):4902-4907.

Nahla, A. M. H. Cancer Associated Thrombosis: Still many unanswered Questions. *Biomed. J. Sci. & Tech. Res.* 2018; 4(3)- 2018. BJSTR. MS.ID.001066. doi: 10.26717/ BJSTR.2018.04.001066 (Nahla 2018).

Quezada, A., Jiménez, D., Bikdeli, B., Muriel, A., Aramberri, M, López-Jiménez, L., Sahuquillo, J. C., Otero, R., Porfidia, A., Monreal, M.; RIETE Investigators. Outcomes after vena cava filter use in patients with cancer-associated venous thromboembolism and contraindications to anticoagulation. *Thromb. Haemost.* 2020; 120: 1035–44.

Roule, V., Verdier, L., Blanchart, K., Ardouin, P., Lemaitre, A., Bignon, M., Sabatier, R., Alexandre, J, Beygui, F. Systematic review and meta-analysis of the prognostic impact of cancer among patients with acute coronary syndrome and/or percutaneous coronary intervention. *BMC Cardiovasc. Disord.* 2020; 20:38.

(2021) NCCN Clinical Practice Guidelines in Oncology (NCCN Guidelines). *Cancer-associated venous thromboembolic disease.* Version 2.2021.

Steffel, J., Collins, R., Antz, M., Cornu, P., Desteghe, L., Haeusler, K. G., Oldgren, J., Reinecke, H., Roldan-Schilling, V., Rowell, N., Sinnaeve, P., Vanassche, T., Potpara, T., Camm, A. J., Heidbüchel, H. 2021 European Heart Rhythm Association practical guide on the use of non-vitamin K antagonist oral anticoagulants in patients with atrial fibrillation. *Europace* 2021;23: 1612–1676.

Sabatino, J., De Rosa, S., Polimeni, A., Sorrentino, S., Indolfi, C. Direct oral anticoagulants in patients with active cancer: a systematic review and meta-analysis. *JACC Cardio Oncol.* 2020; 2:428–440.

Stein, P. D. *Venous thromboembolism in patients with cancer*. In: Stein PD, eds. Pulmonary embolism. 3th ed. John Wiley & Sons Inc.; 2016: Chapter 18:118-127.

Van der Hulle, T., den Exter, P. L., Kooiman, J., van der Hoeven, J. J. M., Huisman, M. V., Kloket, F. A. Meta-analysis of the efficacy and safety of new oral anticoagulants in patients with cancer-associated acute venous thromboembolism. *J. Thromb. Haemost.* 2014; 12: 1116-1120. (Van der Hulle et al., 2014).

Xin, Z., Liu, F., Du, Y., Mao, F., Wang, X., Xu, P., Li, Z., Qian, J., Yao, J. Primary prophylaxis for venous thromboembolism in ambulatory cancer patients: a systematic review and network meta-analysis. *Ann. Cardiothorac. Surg.* 2020; 9:2970–2981.

Yan, Y. D., Ding, Z., Pan, M. M, Xia, Q., Cui, J. J., Wang, L. W., Zhang, C., Gu, Z. C. Net clinical benefit of direct oral anticoagulants in patients with cancer and venous thromboembolism: a systematic review and trade-off analysis. *Front. Cardiovasc. Med.* 2020; 7: 586020.

Chapter 11

Pulmonary Embolism and Pregnancy

Irena Mitevska[1,*], PhD
and Sonja Slinger[2], PhD
[1]University Cardiology Clinic, Medical Faculty, Skopje, North Macedonia
[2]Cardiology Clinic, Clinical Center, Medical Faculty Nis, Serbia

Abstract

Acute pulmonary embolism (PE) remains one of the leading causes of maternal death in high-income countries, resulting in approximately 1.1 mortalities per 100,000 pregnancies, affecting one of 500–3000 cases of pregnant women (Morris et al., 2010). Venous thromboembolism (VTE) risk is 10 times higher in pregnancy, reaching the peak during the postpartum phase, compared to non-pregnant women at a similar age. It is one of the most devastating complications during the pregnancy, urging us to think, screen, and properly treat pregnant women with acute PE. Thromboprophylaxis of patients with previous episodes of deep vein thrombosis (DVT) or PE, or known thrombophilia and other comorbidities that increase PE risk is of great importance in order to ensure safe and healthy pregnancy (James et al., 2006). The baseline pregnancy-related risk increases further in the presence of additional VTE risk factors, including in vitro fertilization during the first trimester, prior VTE, obesity, comorbidities, stillbirth, pre-eclampsia, postpartum bleeding, and cesarean section. Diagnostic radiation exposure in pregnancy should be minimized, and guidelines for the treatment of PE in pregnancy should be strictly followed. This chapter presents the risk factors and latest guidelines-based diagnostic and treatment approaches for acute PE in pregnancy and postpartum periods.

---

* Corresponding Author's Email: peovskai@yahoo.com.

In: Pulmonary Embolism
Editors: Irena Mitevska, Sonja Salinger, Marijan Bosevski et al.
ISBN: 979-8-89113-175-0

Keywords: pregnancy, pulmonary embolism, diagnosis, treatment

Introduction

During pregnancy, VTE can manifest as an isolated lower extremity DVT or as an acute pulmonary embolism. Preventing complications and deaths from PE in pregnancy requires a high index of clinical suspicion focused on fast and accurate diagnosis, which will enable appropriate and on-time initiation of anticoagulation treatment. Clinical diagnosis of pulmonary thromboembolism in pregnancy remains challenging and quite difficult because physiological symptoms and signs that are associated with pregnancy can closely mimic those of PE. Investigations frequently involve radiation exposure both to mother and fetus. Inappropriate care regarding radiation exposure and physician inaction may lead to misdiagnosis and risk to the patient's life (Elgendy et al., 2021). The latest guidelines recommend that in case of clinical suspicion for VTE, treatment can be started while confirmation of a diagnosis is pending (Konstantinides et al., 2021). Diagnosis and timely treatment are crucial for the elimination of potential complications. A clinical team approach, which includes a cardiologist, gynecologist, obstetricians, and anesthesiologist, is necessary to develop an optimal treatment plan in pregnant patients with PE during the pregnancy, delivery, and postpartum phases.

Epidemiology and Risk Factors for Pulmonary Embolism in Pregnancy

Venous thromboembolism complicates 1 in 1000 pregnancies, with much higher prevalence compared to non-pregnant women at similar ages (Marik et al., 2008). Pregnancy is a special phase in a woman's life with increased PE risk, caused by the hypercoagulable state of pregnancy that begins with conception, and increased values of several coagulation factors that do not return to normal until the 8th postpartum week. All three components of "Virchow's triad" which include venous stasis, hypercoagulability, and vascular damage occur during pregnancy and delivery. Pregnancy leads to increased venous stasis in the pelvic and lower limb veins due to the vasodilatory effects of pregnancy hormones and physical obstruction from the gravid uterus. Pregnancy also increases coagulation factors values in preparation for the hemostatic changes in the delivery phase, irrespective of the delivery mode, which itself causes injury of pelvic vessels (Cerneca et al., 1997). More than half of women affected will have had their VTE event by the 20th gestation week (Bremme et al., 2003). DVTs comprise up to 80% of all pregnancy-related VTEs, with a majority of DVTs located in the iliofemoral and pelvic veins, compared to non-pregnant women where the majority of DVTs are popliteofemoral. In pregnant women, the majority of DVTs are left-sided and with iliofemoral distribution, which is partly explained by pelvic compression of the left common iliac vein. Postpartum PE risk increases 20-fold and is assumed to last until the 12th postnatal week, with maximal prevalence in the first postnatal week. (Tepper et al., 2014).

Pregnancy is related to multiple risk factors, and one of the strongest factors are previous pregnancy-related VTE, obesity, multiparity pregnancy, hyperemesis, increased maternal age, thrombophilias, especially homozygous factor V Leiden, and medical morbidities (Sultan et al., 2012). Cesarean section is a strong postnatal risk factor, especially if it is associated with prolonged hospitalization and bed rest, postpartum infection, or bleedings. There are severe procoagulant changes that occur during normal pregnancy, which include reduction of protein S values, increased concentration of factors VII, VIII, vWF and fibrinogen, plasminogen activation inhibitor type 1 (PAI), and prothrombin (Szecsi et al., 2010). Those values start to increase from conception and do not return to baseline values until 8 weeks postpartum. Risk factors for PE in pregnancy are shown in Table 1.

Diagnosis

Normal physiological pregnancy might have symptoms similar to the acute VTE, such as dyspnea, palpitations, and lower extremity swelling that can be difficult to distinguish clinically. It is important to have high clinical suspicion of PE, especially in the case of unilateral gel swelling, sudden dyspnea, tachycardia, or syncope. PE has a wide variety of presenting features, ranging from asymptomatic to shock or sudden death. Several smaller trials suggest that the presenting features in pregnant patients are similar to those reported in PIOPED II (Worsley et al., 1995). The most frequent PE-related symptoms in pregnancy are dyspnea, pleuritic chest pain, cough, sweating, and palpitations.

In pregnant women, it is recommended to use Wells or modified Geneva PE probability scores, which can rule out PE with high sensitivity (Sadeghi et., 2022). Unfortunately, in pregnant women with PE suspicion, diagnosis is established only in 1 of 30 women. Identification of clinically significant PE during pregnancy is challenging, and it is of great importance that clinicians understand the potential for both underdiagnosing and overdiagnosing PE during pregnancy. Imaging is a necessary step to exclude or confirm PE, bearing in mind that D-dimer-based strategies have not been validated in pregnancy (Kline et al., 2005). Lower extremity ultrasound should be used to confirm DVT (Gherman et al., 1999). Computed tomography pulmonary angiography (CTPA) and pulmonary scintigraphy are both recommended modalities.

Table 1. Risk factors for pulmonary embolism in pregnancy

Pre-exiting	Transient	Obstetrics
Previous VTE Heritable/acquired thrombophilia Family history of VTE Medical comorbidities (SLE, nephrotic syndrome, sickle cell disease, cancer, inflammatory conditions) Age >35 years BMI >30 kg·m^{-2} Parity ≥3 Smoking Varicose veins Paraplegia Varicose veins Paraplegia	Early pregnancy Hyperemesis gravidarum Ovarian hyperstimulation syndrome Throughout pregnancy Surgical Procedures (inc. ERPC, postpartum sterilization) Admission Immobility (e.g., symphysis pubis dysfunction) Dehydration Systemic Infection Travel of duration >4 hours	Antenatal Multiple pregnancies Assisted reproduction Therapy Pre-eclampsia Delivery Cesarean section Prolonged labor/Midcavity rotational forceps delivery Postnatal Postpartum hemorrhage (>1 liter) Blood transfusion

VTE- venous thromboembolism, SLE- systemic lupus erythematosus, BMI- body mass index, ERCP-endoscopic retrograde cholangiopancreatography.

Clinical Prediction Rules and D-Dimers

The overall prevalence of confirmed PE in pregnancy is between 2 and 7%. D-dimer values above the threshold for PE 'rule-out' are found in almost 25%

of pregnant women in the third trimester of pregnancy, but also in cases of pre-eclampsia and placental abruption (Chan et al., 2005). Clinical prediction rules used in the non-pregnant population, such as the modified Wells score, are not validated for use in pregnancy due to poor positive predictive values. Still, D-dimer testing with lower limb ultrasound is the focus of diagnostic approaches in normotensive pregnant women with suspected PE and signs of DVT (Damodaram et al., 2009). If there is an intermediate or high pre-test probability, anticoagulation with heparin should be administered before the initiation of diagnostic imaging (Figure 1). If lower limb ultrasound identifies DVT, the diagnosis of PE is indirectly confirmed, taking into consideration the clinical presentation and PE probability. If there is no proximal DVT present or in the case of inconclusive results, a chest X-ray should be performed. In the case of the absence of parenchymal pulmonary abnormalities, the diagnostic pathway should be followed by ventilation/perfusion scintigraphy (V/Q scan), or CTPA, in order to diagnose suspected PE (Gottschalk et al., 2002, Shahir et al., 2010). Arterial oxygen saturation should be measured, and an electrocardiogram conducted in all patients. Electrocardiographic abnormalities are present in approximately 40% of pregnant women with acute PE, including evidence of right bundle branch block, T-wave inversion, and S1Q3T3 pattern.

Concerning the safety of diagnostic procedures in pregnant women, the proposed diagnostic algorithm in patients with suspected PE includes reduction of the anatomical coverage of the scan, reduction of the kilovoltage, using iterative reconstructive techniques, and reducing the contrast-monitoring component of the CTPA (Leung et al., 2011). A normal perfusion scan and a negative CTPA are equally safe for ruling out PE in pregnancy, and the initial choice of diagnostic modality should be determined based on local availability and experience. V/Q SPECT imaging is associated with low fetal and maternal radiation exposure (Chan et al., 2002). Both imaging modalities are associated with a very small increased risk of childhood cancer, with fetal radiation dose related to V/Q scanning slightly higher compared to CTPA (approximately 0.5 mGy and 0.1 mGy, respectively) (Revel et al., 2011). Conventional pulmonary angiography leads to significantly higher radiation exposure to the fetus and should not be used during the pregnancy. Overdiagnosis of PE has potential long-term implications for a pregnant woman, including bleeding risk during delivery, withholding estrogen contraception, and the need for thromboprophylaxis during subsequent pregnancies. Avoiding PE overdiagnosis in pregnancy is similarly important so as not to miss the diagnosis.

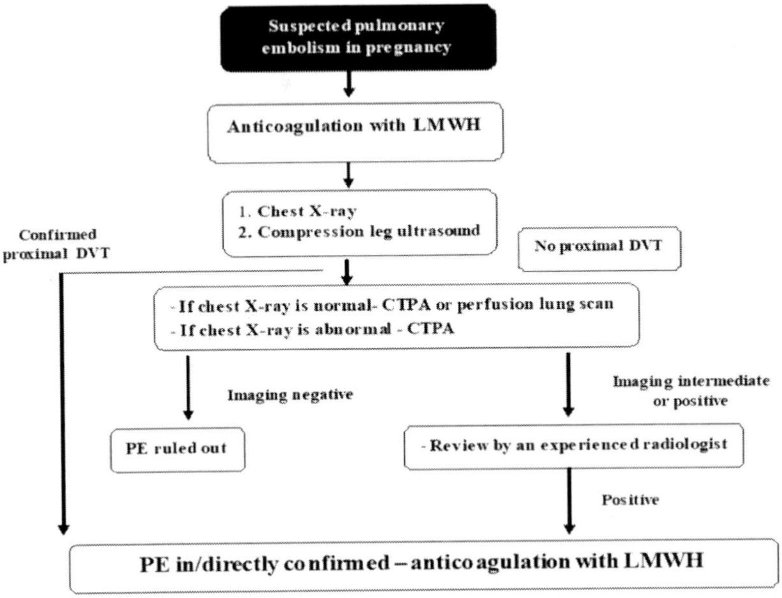

CTPA, computed tomography pulmonary angiography; DVT, deep vein thrombosis; LMWH, low-molecular-weight heparin; PE, pulmonary embolism.

Figure 1. Diagnosis and management of suspected acute PE in pregnancy, modified from Konstantinides et al.

Treatment of Pulmonary Embolism in Pregnancy

High-Risk Unstable Patients with Acute Pulmonary Embolism in Pregnancy

Initial risk stratification is based on an assessment of the patient's hemodynamic status, similarly as in nonpregnant women. Pregnant women have six times higher risk of pulmonary embolism compared to the nonpregnant population at a similar age, with risk peaking during the postpartum period (Nichols et al., 2020). High-risk pulmonary embolism, presenting with hemodynamic instability, is responsible for 10% to 15% of maternal deaths in Europe and North America. All hemodynamically unstable patients with suspected PE have a high risk of death during the first hours and during hospitalization. In hemodynamically unstable patients with high risk of early death, fibrinolytic therapy is linked to a higher bleeding risk. Initiation of heparin anticoagulation is recommended without delay in patients with a high or intermediate clinical probability of PE, while a diagnostic workup is in progress (Regitz-Zagrosek et al., 2018). The European Society of Cardiology (ESC) guidelines on pulmonary embolism and Royal College of Obstetricians and Gynecologists (RCOG) guidelines as well as the American Thoracic and Radiology Society (ATS-STR), and the Society of Thrombosis and Hemostasis (GTH) recommended treatment with empirical therapeutic anticoagulation in patients with hemodynamic instability, while diagnostic workup is ongoing (James et al., 2018). The latest ESC guidelines for the management of acute PE highlight the importance of bedside transthoracic echocardiography in patients with hemodynamic instability. Acute right ventricular (RV) dysfunction can be promptly evaluated, which can potentially explain the hemodynamic deterioration (Konstantinides et al., 2020). Echocardiography can detect other causes of hemodynamic instability, including acute coronary syndrome, cardiac tamponade,aortic dissection, acute valvular dysfunction, or hypovolemia. If PE is indirectly confirmed in all patients with hemodynamic instability, fibrinolytic therapy is recommended in case no absolute contraindications for thrombolysis are present (Blondon et al., 2021). Alternative treatment choices are percutaneous thrombectomy or catheter thrombolysis. However, scientific data reported that only one-third of high-risk unstable pregnant women with PE received thrombolytic treatment (Bates et al., 2018). Treatment decision regarding this very vulnerable patient population should be individualized case by case, taking into account the clinical presentation and the patient's overall risk. Half a dose of tPA (50 mg) was equally effective compared to standard recommended dose of 100 mg over 2 hours. A systematic review, which included 127 intermediate and high-risk PE pregnant women treated with thrombolysis, thrombectomy, or ECMO, reported survival rates of 94 and 86% following thrombolysis and surgical thrombectomy, respectively (Martillotti et al., 2017). After thrombolysis, major bleeding was reported in 18% and 58% during pregnancy and in the postpartum period, respectively. During the peripartum and postpartum period, systemic thrombolysis treatment carries an extremely high risk of bleeding, and in these situations, other advanced therapies should also be evaluated as fast treatment options.

Stable Patients with Acute Pulmonary Embolism in Pregnancy

Low-molecular-weight heparin (LMWH) is the treatment of choice in clinically stable pregnant women with PE, having more predictable pharmacokinetics and a more favorable risk profile (Couturaud et al., 2001). Based on the efficacy of data from trials in the non-pregnant population, LMWH is more effective than unfractionated heparin (UFH) and is associated with lower mortality and a lower risk of bleeding. LMWH does not cross the placenta in contrast to direct oral anticoagulants (DOACs) and vitamin K antagonists (VKAs), and does not present a risk of fetal teratogenicity or hemorrhage (Lepercq et al., 2001). Consequently, coumarins should be avoided in pregnancy apart from the high-risk cases, such as women with articificial heart valves, in whom they have been used after embryogenesis in the first trimester. The use of VKAs in the third trimester can result in fetal and neonatal hemorrhage, central nervous system anomalies, as well as placental abruption. Fondaparinux has been used in pregnancy, and safety data suggests that it is suitable, but it is generally only prescribed in cases of severe heparin allergy or heparin-induced thrombocytopenia. LMWH is generally safe and easy to use with either once-a-day or twice-a-day dosing (1 mg/kg twice daily, or 1.5 mg/k once daily). Regular APTT monitoring is unnecessary in most patients (Wiegers et al., 2020), which can be technically challenging due to potential heparin resistance. Anti-activated coagulation factor X monitoring may be used in specific high-risk situations, including reduced renal function, recurrent VTE, and severe differences in body weight (less than 50 kg or greater than 90 kg). The risk for heparin-induced thrombocytopenia with LMWH is also very low. DOACs are contraindicated in pregnant patients; however, they can be used postnatally if the woman is not breastfeeding. DOACs cross the placenta, and they elevate the risk of anomalies, hemorrhage, and embryopathies, as shown in the results of animal studies. Anticoagulation medications type and safety use in pregnancy are shown in Table 2.

Anticoagulation Therapy During Labor and Delivery

Management of delivery, including the type of anesthesia requires a multidisciplinary approach and planned delivery to reduce the risk of spontaneous labor while the patient is on full anticoagulation treatment (Table

3). Delivery planning involves the balance between the postpartum bleeding risk in a woman on full therapeutic anticoagulation with the risk of worsening or recurrent PE when treatment is stopped during the induction of labor process. If regional analgesia is planned to be used in women treated with therapeutic LMWH doses, over 24 h should have passed from the last LMWH dose before insertion of a spinal or epidural needle in patients with normal renal function, without extreme body weight values (Table 3). In patients with recent PE, LMWH should be converted to unfractionated heparin (UFH) over 36 hours prior to delivery, and infusion should be stopped 4 – 6 h prior to planned delivery, with activated partial thromboplastin time in normal values prior to regional anesthesia (Wiegers et al., 2020). Timing of reinitiation of LMWH after delivery will depend upon the delivery mode and the assessment of thrombotic vs. bleeding risk. LMWH should not be reintroduced for minimum 4 hours after removal of the epidural catheter. Anticoagulant treatment should be used for over 6 weeks after delivery and with a minimum overall treatment duration of 3 months. LMWH and warfarin can be applied to breastfeeding mothers, while the use of DOACs is not recommended. Lower doses of LMWH should be prescribed in women with renal failure and creatinine clearance <30 mL·min−1. It is reasonable to continue therapeutic anticoagulation 6–12 h after vaginal delivery and 12–24 h following cesarean section and once hemostasis has been achieved. Prevention of pulmonary embolism with LMWH is indicated during pregnancy and in all postpartum women with a history of previous VTE, which is described in more detail in Chapter 7.

Table 2. Safety of anticoagulant use in pregnancy

Anticoagulant type	Safety and use in pregnancy
LMWH	Enoxaparin, Daltaparin; dose 1 mg/kg BID, does not cross the placenta, anticoagulation of choice in pregnancy; may need to adjust dose with increasing weight/may need to monitor anti-Xa levels (goal 0.5–1.1 U/mL).
UFH	May be used in place of LMWH in renal failure, high-risk PE, during delivery, it has a short half-life; IV infusion or injections; need to monitor anti-Xa levels - volume of distribution / weight changes during pregnancy.

Table 2. (Continued)

Anticoagulant type	Safety and use in pregnancy
NOACS	Clinical trials with NOACs excluded pregnant women. Association with congenital anomalies, bleeding, implantation failure in animal studies.
VKA	Warfarin crosses the placenta and has teratogenic effects; up to 6.4% risk of congenital abnormalities, risk of fetal hemorrhage after organogenesis. Should not be used for treatment of VTE in pregnancy.
Synthetic heparins	Fondaparinux is not thought to increase risk of congenital malformations. Small amounts cross the placenta, with measurable effect on neonatal anti-Xa levels. Clinical significance of placental transfer is unknown.
Thrombin inhibitors	Lepirudin is not expected to increase the risk of congenital anomalies. Human case reports and animal studies do not show evidence of malformation. Lepirudin does cross the rat placenta. Argatroban use in animal studies at doses lower than human doses. Rare case reports do not show evidence of congenital anomalies; safety cannot be ascertained. It has been used in patients with HIT and heparin allergy.

Abbreviations: BID, twice daily; HIT, heparin-induced thrombocytopenia; IV, intravenous; LMWH, low molecular weight heparins; NOAC/DOAC, novel/direct anticoagulants; PE, pulmonary embolism; UFH, unfractionated heparins; VKA, vitamin K antagonists; VTE, venous thromboembolism.

Table 3. Management of anticoagulation therapy around labor and delivery period

Gestational Age at Time of PE	Treatment plan
< 2 weeks before labor	Treat with intravenous heparin or place an IVC filter (preferably retrievable) and consider induction. Restart anticoagulation with LMWH or UFH postpartum and plan for removal of IVC filter.
2–4 weeks before labor	Treat initially with LMWH and consider switching to IV heparin at approximately

Gestational Age at Time of PE	Treatment plan
	38 weeks of gestation in consultation with the obstetric team for a planned induction. Stop IV heparin 6 h before anticipated delivery.
More than 1 month before labor	Depending on patient's risk for fast labor may continue LMWH until planned induction or consider switching from LMWH to UFH at term and follow with anti-Xa levels.
Recommendations for all women on anticoagulation during pregnancy	Patients should be instructed to stop heparin injections at the first sign of labor. Therapeutic LMWH should be discontinued at least 24 h before regional anesthesia or planned delivery. LMWH should not be restarted for 4 h after the use of regional anesthesia or after the epidural catheter has been removed. The epidural catheter should not be removed within 12 h of the most recent injection of LMWH.

Abbreviations: IV, intravenous; IVC, inferior vena cava filter; LMWH, low molecular weight heparin; UFH, unfractionated heparin; VTE, venous thromboembolism.

Inferior Vena Cava Filters

There is a specific role for inferior vena cava (IVC) filters in the management of acute PTE in pregnancy. However, because of the risks associated with insertion and removal, which include a fatality rate of 0.1–0.3%, filter migration, filter fracture, and IVC perforation in 5% of patients, their use is limited. When required, a temporary cava filter (retrievable IVC filter) may be used in women who are delivering or are expected to deliver having less than 2 weeks of anticoagulation, a history of recurrent VTE despite adequate anticoagulation treatment, or in women where anticoagulation is contraindicated (Gupta et al., 2008).

Management of Postpartum Period

VTE management in the postpartum period includes the use of LMWH or warfarin, which are proven safe in breastfeeding women, and DOACS in non-breastfeeding women. Therapy should be continued for at least 6 weeks postnatal and for a minimum of 3 months in total. The ongoing risk of thrombosis should be assessed, including past personal and family history, and possible thrombophilia screening is also advised. Management of any future pregnancies should also be discussed, which usually involves the use of prophylactic LMWH from conception until at least 6 weeks of the postnatal period (Middeldorp et al., 2011).

Conclusion

Guidelines and recommendations on the diagnosis and treatment of PE in pregnancy should be followed when making individual treatment decisions. Assessment of PE probability, fast diagnosis with proper management, and risk assessment are necessary in order to reduce major complications and catastrophic outcomes. The use of noninvasive imaging, especially echocardiography, is important for PE diagnosis and risk stratification. Immediate reperfusion with thrombolysis, surgical embolectomy, catheter-directed low-dose thrombolysis, or percutaneous thrombectomy should be applied in high-risk patients. LMWH is a drug of choice in stable patients for thromboprophylaxis and acute PE treatment. The peripartum and postpartum periods are extremely vulnerable to pulmonary embolism management, so a multidisciplinary team of experts in PE treatment in pregnancy should be consulted in order to reach a consensus on the best individual treatment approach.

References

Bates, S. M., Rajasekhar, A., Middeldorp, S., McLintock, C., Rodger, M. A., James, A. H., Vazquez, S. R., Greer, I. A. Riva, J. J., Bhatt, M., Schwab, N., Barrett, D., LaHaye, A., Rochwerg, B. American Society of Hematology 2018 guidelines for management of venous thromboembolism: venous thromboembolism in the context of pregnancy. *Blood Adv.* 2018 Nov 27; 2(22): 3317–3359.

Blondon, M., Martinez, de Tejada, B., Glauser, F., Righini, M., Robert-Ebadi, H. Management of high-risk pulmonary embolism in pregnancy. *Thromb Res.* 2021; 204:57-65.

Bremme, K. A., Haemostatic changes in pregnancy. *Best Pract. Res. Clin. Haematol.* 2003Jun; 16(2):153-68.

Cerneca, F., Ricci, G., Simeone, R., Malisano, M., Alberico, S., Guaschino, S. Coagulation and fibrinolysis changes in normal pregnancy. Increased levels of procoagulants and reduced levels of inhibitors during pregnancy induce a hypercoagulable state, combined with a reactive fibrinolysis. European Journal of Obstetrics and Gynecology and Reproductive Biology. *Eur. J. Obstet. Gynecol. Reprod. Biol.,*1997 May;73(1):31-6.

Chan, W. S., Ray, J. G., Murray, S., Coady, G. E., Coates, G., Ginsberg, J. S. Suspected pulmonary embolism in pregnancy: clinical presentation, results of lung scanning, and subsequent maternal and pediatric outcomes. *Arch. Intern. Med.* 2002; 162: 1170–1175.

Couturaud, F., Julian, J. A., Kearon, C. Low molecular weight heparin administered once versus twice daily in patients with venous thromboembolism: a meta-analysis. *Thromb. Haemost.* 2001;86:980–4,

Damodaram, M., Kaladindi, M., Luckit, J., Yoong, W. D-dimers as a screening test for venous thromboembolism in pregnancy: is it of any use? *J. Obstet. Gynaecol.* 2009; 29:101,

Elgendy, I. Y., Gad, M. M., Mansoor, H., Mahmoud, A. N., Elbadawi, A., Saad, A., Saad, M., Elkaryoni, A., Secemsky, E.A., Mamas, M.A., Monreal, M., Weinberg, I., Pepine, C.J. Acute Pulmonary Embolism During Pregnancy and Puerperium: National Trends and In-Hospital Outcomes. *Mayo Clin. Proc.* 2021; 96:2102.

Gherman, R. B., Goodwin, T. M., Leung, B., Byrne, J. D., Hethumumi, R., Montoro, M. Incidence, clinical characteristics, and timing of objectively diagnosed venous thromboembolism during pregnancy. *Obstet. Gynecol.* 1999; 94:730.

Gottschalk, A., Stein, P. D., Goodman, L. R., Sostman, H. D. Overview of Prospective Investigation of Pulmonary Embolism Diagnosis II. *Semin. Nucl. Med.* 2002; 32:173.

Gupta, S., Ettles, D. F., Robinson, G. J., Lidow, S. V. Inferior vena cava filter use in pregnancy: preliminary experience. *BJOG* 2008;115:785–8.

James, A., Birsner, M., Kaimal, A. ACOG Practice Bulletin No. 196: Thromboembolism in Pregnancy. American College of Obstetricians and Gynecologists' Committee on Practice Bulletins-Obstetrics. *Obstet. Gynecol.* 2018 Jul;132(1): e1-e17.

James, A. H., Jamison, M. G., Brancazio, L. R., Myers, E. R. Venous thromboembolism during pregnancy and the postpartum period: incidence, risk factors, and mortality. *Am. J. Obstet. Gynecol.* 2006; 194:1311.

Kline, J. A., Williams, G. W., Hernandez-Nino, J. D-dimer concentrations in normal pregnancy: new diagnostic thresholds are needed. *Clin. Chem.* 2005; 51:825.

Konstantinides, S. V., Meyer, G., Becattini, C., Bueno, H., Geersing, G. J., Harjola, V. P., Huisman, M. V., Humbert, M., Jennings, C. S., Jiménez, D., Kucher, N., Lang, I. M., Lankeit, M., Lorusso, R., Mazzolai, L., Meneveau, N., Áinle, F. N., Prandoni, P., Pruszczyk, P., Righini, M., Torbicki, A., Belle, E.V., Zamorano, J. L.; ESC Scientific Document Group. ESC Guidelines for the diagnosis and management of acute pulmonary embolism developed in collaboration with the European Respiratory Society (ERS). *Eur Heart J.* 2020 Jan 21;41(4):543-603.

Kovac, M., Mikovic, Z., Rakicevic, L., Srzentic, S., Mandic, V., Djordjevic, V., Radojkovic, D., Elezovic, I. The use of D-dimer with new cutoff can be useful in diagnosis of venous thromboembolism in pregnancy. *Eur. J. Obstet. Gynecol. Reprod. Biol.* 2010; 148:27.

Lepercq, J., Conard, J., Borel-Derlon, A., Darmon, J. Y., Boudignat, O., Francoual, C., Priollet, P., Cohen, C., Yvelin, N., Schved, J. F., Tournaire, M., Borg, J. Y. Venous thromboembolism during pregnancy: a retrospective study of enoxaparin safety in 624 pregnancies. *BJOG* 2001; 108:1134–40.

Leung, A. N., Bull, T. M., Jaeschke, R., Lockwood, C. J., Boiselle, P. M., Hurwitz, L. M., James, A. H., McCullough L. B., Menda. Y, Paidas, M. J., Royal, H. D., Tapson, V. F., Winer-Muram, H. T., Chervenak, F.A., Cody, D. D., McNitt-Gray, M. F., Stave, C. D., and Tuttle, B. D. on behalf of the ATS/STR Committee on Pulmonary Embolism in Pregnancy ATS/STR Committee on Pulmonary Embolism in Pregnancy. An official American Thoracic Society/Society of Thoracic Radiology clinical practice guideline: evaluation of suspected pulmonary embolism in pregnancy. *Am. J. Respir. Crit. Care Med.* 2011; 184:1200.

Marik, P. E., Plante, L. A. Venous thromboembolic disease and pregnancy. *N. Engl. J. Med.* 2008; 359:2025.

Martillotti, G., Boehlen, F., Robert-Ebadi, H., Jastrow, N., Righini, M., M Blondon, M. Treatment options for severe pulmonary embolism during pregnancy and the postpartum period: a systematic review. *J. Thromb. Haemost*, 2017. 15(10): p. 1942–1950.

Middeldorp, S. How I treat pregnancy-related venous thromboembolism. *Blood* 2011; 118:5394-400.

Morris, J. M., Algert, C. S., Roberts, C. L. Incidence and risk factors for pulmonary embolism in the postpartum period. *J. Thromb. Haemost.* 2010; 8:998.

Nichols, K.M., Henkin, S., Creager, M.A. Venous thromboembolism associated with pregnancy: JACC Focus Seminar. *J. Am. Coll. Cardiol.* 2020;76: 2128-2141.

Regitz-Zagrosek, V., Roos-Hesselink, J. W., Bauersachs, J., Blomström-Lundqvist, C., Cífková, R., Bonis, M. D., Iung, B., Johnson, M. R., Kintscher, U., Kranke, P., Lang, I. M., Morais, J., Pieper, P. G., Presbitero, P., Price, S., Rosano, G. M., Seeland, U., Simoncini, T., Swan, L., Warnes, C. A.; ESC Scientific Document Group. 2018 ESC guidelines for the management of cardiovascular diseases during pregnancy. *Eur. Heart J.* 2018;39: 3165-3241.

Revel, M. P., Cohen, S., Sanchez, O., Collignon, M. A., Thiam, R., Redheuil, A., Meyer, G., Frija, G. Pulmonary embolism during pregnancy: diagnosis with lung scintigraphy or CT angiography? *Radiology* 2011; 258:590.

Sadeghi, S., Bahrami, P., Far, S. K., Arabi, Z. Determining the diagnostic value of three clinical criteria Wells', YEARS and modified Geneva in pregnant women with suspected pulmonary thromboembolism. *Am J Cardiovasc Dis.* 2022; 12(4): 240–246.

Shahir, K., Goodman, L. R., Tali, A., Thorsen, K. M., Hellman, R. S. Pulmonary embolism in pregnancy: CT pulmonary angiography versus perfusion scanning. *AJR Am. J. Roentgenol.* 2010; 195:W214.

Sultan, A. A., West, J., Tata, L. J., Fleming, K. M., Nelson-Piercy, C., Grainge, M. J. Risk of first venous thromboembolism in and around pregnancy: a population-based cohort study. *Br. J. Haematol.* (2012) 156:366–73.

Szecsi, P. B., Jørgensen, M., Klajnbard, A., Andersen, M. R., Colov, N. P., Stender, S. Haemostatic reference intervals in pregnancy. *Thromb Haemost.* 2010;103: 718–27.

Tepper, N. K., Boulet, S. L., Whiteman, M. K., Monsour, M., Marchbanks, P.A., Hooper, W.C., Curtis, K.M. Postpartum venous thromboembolism: incidence and risk factors. *Obstet. Gynecol.* 2014 May;123(5):987-996.

Wiegers, H. M. and Middeldorp, S. Contemporary best practice in the management of pulmonary embolism during pregnancy. *Ther. Adv. Respir. Dis.* 2020 Jan-Dec; 14: 1753466620914222.

Worsley, D.F ., Alavi, A. Comprehensive analysis of the results of the PIOPED Study. Prospective Investigation of Pulmonary Embolism Diagnosis Study. *J. Nucl. Med.* 1995 Dec; 36(12):2380-7.

Chapter 12

Regional Registry of Acute Pulmonary Embolism: Organization, Aims, and Achievements

Slobodan Obradovic[1,2,*], PhD
Boris Dzudovic[2,3], PhD
Jovan Matijasevic[4,5], PhD
Sonja Salinger[6], PhD
and Irena Mitevska[7], PhD

[1]Clinic of Cardiology, Military Medical Academy, Belgrade, Serbia
[2]School of Medicine, University of Defense, Belgrade, Serbia
[3]School of Medicine, University of Defense, Belgrade, Serbia, Clinic of Emergency Internal Medicine, Military Medical Academy, Belgrade, Serbia
[4]School of Medicine, University of Defense, Belgrade, Serbia
[5]School of Medicine, University of Novi Sad, Serbia
[6]Clinic of Cardiology, Clinical Center Nis, University of Nis, Serbia
[7]UniversityCardiology Clinic, School of Medicine, University "St Cyril and Methodius" Skopje, North Macedonia

Abstract

Acute pulmonary embolism is a very heterogeneous disease; in fact, potential causes are extremely different and this can influence the treatment and prognosis of the patients. However, the hemodynamic state, which depends of the size of pulmonary artery obstruction and previous cardio-pulmonary status, is the main prognostic factor for survival. Patients with hypotension due to PE have a high risk of adverse

* Corresponding Author's Email: sloba.d.obradovic@gmail.com.

In: Pulmonary Embolism
Editors: Irena Mitevska, Sonja Salinger, Marijan Bosevski et al.
ISBN: 979-8-89113-175-0

outcomes. Secondly, the patient may be normotensive but with severe right ventricle dysfunction, and these patients are at the crossroad and can deteriorate or further stabilize. Unfortunately, randomized trials did not solve the problem of whether patients with intermediate-high-risk PE should be re-perfused and how. Estimation of risk of bleeding is also very important because anticoagulant and thrombolytic therapy are the main drugs for the treatment of acute PE, and both can cause severe bleeding. Since there are many unresolved, very important clinical questions in acute PE management, the role of large, carefully created and conducted registries with a high number of patients could be very useful in resolving many problematic issues. Therefore, we created the local registry of acute PE patients, containing a prospective collection of carefully chosen medical data with the aim of resolving some important clinical questions. Should we, when, and how, re-perfuse intermediate-high risk PE patients? Do we need some fine-tuned risk stratification? How do we estimate the risk of bleeding with or without thrombolytic therapy? When do we discharge patients, not only low-risk patients, but also intermediate- and high-risk patients? In this work, we decided to generate the local acute PE registry and, through the clustering of variables, cover some important issues, aiming to resolve some clinical problems in the management of acute PE which stand before us. We founded the Regional PE registry in 2011 as a single-center registry. From 2015, five university centers and one big regional hospital from Serbia, and university centers from Banja Luka, Bosnia and Herzegovina, Podgorica Montenegro, and Skopje North Macedonia joined the registry. The positive finding on the computed tomography pulmonary angiography (CTPA) and the symptoms of PE lasting no longer the 14 days are the main inclusion criteria for participation in the registry. In the period of 12 days, 1,815 patients were enrolled. During this period, 15 manuscripts were published in extenso, and several abstracts were presented in international scientific meetings. Using data from the registry, we succeeded in expanding our knowledge about risk stratification, estimation of bleeding risk, and to improve the protocols for treatment of acute PE.

Keywords: pulmonary embolism, registry, treatment, risk stratification, bleeding

Introduction

Data from the large multicenter registries are very important to study all aspects of the investigated diseases. Randomized trials (RT) always have many inclusion and exclusion criteria, which means that the data from the RT have limited generalizability; however, the quality of data is very reliable because of the careful, prospective data collection and precise definition of many variables used. On the other side, although many registries are prospectively guided, the focuses of investigation are often created after the data collection, and the nature of the investigation is actually retrospective with many pitfalls considering, imprecise variable definitions, and many potential biases, especially in patients where the collection of data are difficult, like high risk-patients, neurology-psychiatry patients, or patients with advanced malignancy where there are ethical and technical problems to rich the data.

Several registries of acute pulmonary embolism patients published very important data about the clinical features of the disease, including risk stratification, outcome, and characteristics of some special subgroups of patients. Some of the main papers from the registries are presented in Table 1. It is important to know that the many important results are very different in various registries, and it is very important to standardize at least some of the pivotal variables, especially outcomes, such as all-cause, and PE-related death, bleeding, recurrent diseases, late complications, among others. Accordingly, it is important to use standardized definitions created by the scientific associations, e.g., definition of pulmonary-related death and classification of the cause of death in patients with venous thromboembolism suggested by the International Society of Thrombosis and Hemostasis (ISTH) (Trithcler et al., 2020), or definition of major and clinically relevant non-major bleeding by the same association (Schulman S et al., 2005 and 2010).

Some of the most important registries of acute PE patients are presented briefly in Table 1 (Monreal et al., 2022; Goldhaber et al., 1999; Cazzaca et al., 2012; Zhang et al., 2022; Yamashita et al., 2020; Chopard et al., 2019). The largest, and certainly the most productive one is the RIETE registry (Monreal et al., 2022), with a large number of qualitative publications in various areas of acute PE management.

Every registry has started with some purpose, and sometimes, the purpose is limited to the investigation of a relatively small area of interest, and sometimes registries designed as a large "fishing net" to catch different and often unplanned scientific data and to solve some important issues. Both approaches have their advantages and disadvantages; hence, a registry is created with many tasks, very often you cannot go deep enough for some particular problem, or conversely if a more focused registry is created, it is possible to neglect some important confounding factor rendering to certain biases.

Table 1. Some of the most important registries regarding acute PE

Registry	Approximate number of PE patients enrolled in the latest publication	Main fields of investigation
RIETE (Registro Informatizado de Pacientes con Enfermedad TromboEmbolica)	38,000 patients	Risk stratification, bleeding on anticoagulation therapy, many subgroup analyses in respect of risk stratification and different outcomes, analysis of various therapeutic approaches
ICOPER (International Cooperative Pulmonary Embolism Registry)	2,500	Clinical presentation, risk stratification, therapeutic approach, echocardiography and outcome
IPER (Italian Pulmonary Embolism Registry)	1,700	Risk stratification, echocardiography and outcome
CURES (China pUlmonary Thromboembolism REgistry Study (CURES) Investigators)	7,400	Outcomes with respect to some characteristics of patients at presentation
COMMAND VTE (JAPAN acute VTE registry)	1,700	Validation of sPESI score
FRENCH registry	1,100	Use of oral anticoagulants

The Regional Pulmonary Embolism Registry (REPER)

The military medical academy was the founder of the Regional PE Registry (REPER). In the period of 2015–2022, five university clinics and one general hospital from Serbia and university cardiology clinics from Banja Luka (Bosnia and Herzegovina), Podgorica (Montenegro), and Skopje (North Macedonia) are involved in the registry. All patients have at least a segmental pulmonary embolism. We insisted that all patients have echocardiography assessment and biomarker measurement at admission. We encourage the use of thrombolytic therapy in high-risk patients and in intermediate-high-risk PE patients who did not improve after the first 24 hours of anticoagulant therapy. Meticulous assessment of bleeding risk was performed from the beginning of the REPER. We also aim to investigate potential easily usable ECG markers for the estimation of the success of therapy in the relief of the right ventricle overload.

Special attention was given to comorbidities and their impact on outcomes and adverse events. Oncology and cardiovascular patients were in focus since the treatments and the stages of this disease are very important to the management of acute PE.

Gender-related differences are also in focus of our investigation. We believe that RV function in women is more sensible to acute overload by the obstruction of the pulmonary artery tree, and the imaging procedures and their parameters should be adjusted for gender.

Several clinical issues were aroused by the physicians who lead the REPER, and some of them are presented here.

Improvement of the Risk Stratification

Heart failure with reduced ejection fraction (HFrEF) was presented as 5%, mildly reduced ejection fraction was presented as 4%, and HF with preserved EF was presented in 9% of the patients. We revealed that patients with HF had higher in-hospital mortality, and this is especially pronounced in patients with HFrEF who had increased mortality regardless of the initial risk assessment (Obradovic et al., 2020). Renal function at admission was also investigated in our registry (Salinger-Martinovic et al., 2020). We think that a decrease in glomerular filtration rate, either as chronic renal failure or as an acute renal failure, contributes significantly to the outcome of acute PE, and the addition of this parameter improves the prognostic value of simplified Pulmonary Embolism Score Index (sPESI) and European Society of Cardiology model of risk stratification.

In the treatment of acute ST-elevation myocardial infarction, ST segment resolution is a very important sign of myocardial tissue reperfusion and correlates with survival and left ventricle function. Accordingly, as acute PE can cause severe RV stretching with acute electrocardiography (ECG) changes, we were looking for the ECG signs which could be used as a guide in the treatment of acute PE like we use ST-segment resolution in acute STEMI. We discovered that S wave resolution in DI and especially in a VL standard lead, could be useful for that purpose (Novicic et al., 2019). Early S-wave resolution, even in patients with high-risk PE was associated with low mortality and success of reperfusion (Novicic et al., 2020).

According to our data, there are several important differences between women and men regarding the prognostic significance of symptoms and several laboratory and imaging variables. Thus, we found that syncope at presentation was associated with increased mortality in women but not in men (Dzudovic et al., 2020). Furthermore, tachycardia at admission has had a negative predictive value for early death only in women (Matijasevic et al., 2021).

Gender, age, body mass index, and severity of PE can importantly modify the clinical presentation of acute PE, and it is crucial for the diagnostic workup to be aware of these relationships (Ruzicic et al., 2023).

Embolization of the thrombi is one of the crucial dismal processes in venous thrombosis. Some patients are prone to embolization, and some of them are not. We have found that the presence of symptomatic leg deep vein thrombosis in patients with intermediate-high-risk PE had a better prognosis than patients without (Obradovic et al., 2022). We also found that patients with intermediate-high risk PE and symptomatic DVT did not have an excess of recurrent PE with the use of thrombolytic therapy (Obradovic et al., 2022).

Use of Biomarkers for Risk Stratification in PE

Two groups of the most important biomarkers are used for the risk stratification of PE patients, cardiac troponins (cTn) and brain natriuretic peptides (BNP). However, we think that these two groups of markers might have some different predictive values with respect to age and comorbidities. It is also important to differentiate between quantitative and qualitative predictive values of these parameters as well as do we want to predict all-cause or PE-related death. If we use these markers as "positive or negative," both of them have very good negative predictive value, but if we use them as continuous variables, it seems that BNP has much better sensitivity for the prediction of PE-related death in various subgroups of patients (Jovanovic et al., 2019; Jovanovic et al., 2021). The use of troponins as the only biomarker for the risk stratification in intermediate-risk PE, may lead to an overestimation of risk in elderly patients, and the opposite underestimation of risk in younger patients.

Admission glycemia was a well-studied parameter for various acute states in cardiovascular patients. We have found that admission glycemia is more important for the risk prediction in diabetic than in non-diabetic patients (Jovanovic et al., 2022). It will be important to study if the quality of diabetes treatment influences an outcome in acute PE patients.

Hemostasis Parameters in Acute PE

Pulmonary embolism is a consequence of venous thrombosis and embolization, which means that the balances between coagulation, anticoagulation, and fibrinolysis are the main pathophysiology of the disease. We assumed that large venous thrombosis and embolism of the large thrombi into the pulmonary arteries are a kind of consumable coagulopathy. Hence, our data confirmed that patients with severe PE had lower levels of antithrombin, protein C, and coagulation factor VII, which are also associated with higher in-hospital mortality (Dzudovic et al., 2021; Dzudovic et al., 2022).

Inflammation in PE

Systemic inflammatory response correlate to the severity of PE, and patients with secondary pneumonia or pulmonary infarctions had also higher blood levels of C reactive protein. We have shown that blood CRP level in patients with spontaneous PE was associated with higher hospital mortality (Milic et al., 2018; Milic et al., 2019).

Estimation of Bleeding Risk in PE

The algorithm for the treatment of PE patients is oriented only to the mortality risk, and the main treatment options are thrombolytic therapy and anticoagulant therapy, which carry significant risk for bleeding. There is only one large randomized trial considering the use of thrombolytics in intermediate-high risk PE. This study caused confusion in the treatment of this important group of patients. Although it was a positive trial, where tenecteplase (TNK) reduced the primary end-point, which was the composite of death and hemodynamic deterioration in the 7 days, major bleeding exceeded 11% and intracranial bleeding 2%, which points out the importance of safety issues. The result of this was to change the recommendation of using reperfusion therapy of any kind in this subgroup of patients from class IIb (might be considered) to class III (not recommended), which means that this kind of therapy resulted in more harm than benefit which could probably cost life a thousand of patients in the future with low bleeding risk who are on the hemodynamic edge and who need thrombolytic therapy in the real world. The use of TNK in the full dose, like using ST-segment elevation in myocardial infarction (STEMI), was not a good idea from the beginning, especially when the inclusion criteria for the PEITHO study (Meyer et al., 2015) favored enrollment of older patients. Patients with intermediate-high risk PE do not need bolus, high-dose thrombolytic therapy at admission to the hospital. They need some time for evaluation because 90% of these patients go well with anticoagulant therapy alone. It is obvious that we need some more sophisticated methods for risk stratification in these patients, especially during the first 24–48 hours from admission. On the other side, assessment of bleeding risk on thrombolysis is very important, and it is not recognized as a treatment option modulator. We validated the Pulmonary Embolism Bleeding Score Index (PEBSI) for the prediction of bleeding on t-PA-based thrombolytic therapy (Obradovic et al., 2022), and according to them, patients could be divided into low- and high-risk bleeding risk. This score is only the first step for using a bleeding risk assessment for the treatment modulation in intermediate-high risk PE.

Catheter-Directed Therapy in Acute Pulmonary Embolism

The place of catheter-directed therapy (CDT) is not defined in the current guidelines. It is recommended in high-risk patients who cannot be treated with systemic thrombolysis or in other patients' risk groups when they deteriorate. However, CDT was not tested by the randomized studies, which had hard end-point clinical outcomes in neither of these indications. Mechanical CDT, using aspiration and fragmentation of thrombi, might be a good option for patients who have very high risk for bleeding and who need prompt decrease of pulmonary arteries obstruction. In this case, we are dealing with a life-threatening situation and with very large burden of thrombotic mass. Large-diameter aspiration catheters are designed for this purpose, and are probably the future for this kind of devices (Pruszczyk et al., 2022). However, low-dose tPA therapy through the various catheters could be a valuable option for intermediate-high-risk patients with some additional risk factors for deterioration. In a few hours, in this way, locally driven very small amount of tPA could be sufficient to relieve the RV overload and stabilize the threatening situation. However, in both of these approaches we need a cath-lab and an experienced team who can perform these interventions.

Catheter-directed therapy is in the beginning in Serbia, although the first interventions in sub-acute PE patients were described in 2003 (Obradovic et al., 2011). The series of intermediate/high-risk PE patients treated with ultrasound-facilitated thrombolysis from 2013–2019 in the Military Medical Academy Belgrade, was presented in 2019 (Sekulic et al., 2019; Sekulic et al., 2019). This therapy had a very low risk of dying and relatively low systemic bleeding risk but a high risk of bleeding in the place of vascular access.

We planned a randomized trial using a registry net using low-dose infusion of tPA for intermediate-high-risk PE patients who had some additional risk factors.

Direct Oral Anticoagulants (DOAC) and Hemostasis Changes Under Them

We were interested in how different coagulation and anticoagulation factors are affected by the use of different DOACs. We measured these factors before the next dose of the drug after one month of therapy or acute PE. We have found higher activity of coagulation factors under apixaban compared to rivaroxaban and dabigatran, with similar d-dimer levels (Dzudovic et al., 2019; Dzudovic et al., 2023). This finding could explain why patients on apixaban had the lowest bleeding risk and higher thrombotic risk when we decreased the dose of apixaban. Our group also developed the original high-performance liquid chromatography method for the measurement of apixaban blood concentrations (Dzudovic et al., 2022).

Conclusion

Since there were only a few large randomized trials in acute PE, there are a lot of questions in front of the physicians who deal with this disease. There is no such cardiovascular disease where registries were very important for the many scientific steps which have been performed in the last decades. The involvement in the large, well-organized registry very much improves the organization and treatment of patients with pulmonary embolism in hospitals who were involved, and the benefit for the patients is achieved for the participating patients. Sharing of experience and data is very important for going forward in this field, and the registries are one of the best tools for that.

References

Casazza, F., Becattini, C., Bongarzoni, A., Cuccia, C., Roncon, L., Favretto, G., Zonzin, P., Pignataro, L., Agnelli, G. Clinical features and short-term outcomes of patients with acute pulmonary embolism. *The Italian Pulmonary Embolism Registry (IPER) Multicenter Study Thromb Res* (2012) 130(6):847-852.

Chopard, R., Andarelli, J. N., Humbert, S., Falvo, N., Morel-Aleton, M., Bonnet, B., Napporn, G., Kalbacher, K., Obert, L., Degano, B., Cappelier, G.,Cottin, Y., Schiele, F., Meneveau. N. Prescription patterns of direct oral anticoagulants in pulmonary embolism: A prospective multicenter French registry. *Thromb Res.* (2019) 174:27-33.

Dzudovic, B. Predictive value of the activity of haemostasis factors measured in the early phase of acute pulmonary embolism for hospital mortality. *Doctor thesis, Military Medical Academy,* School of Medicine, University of Defense, Belgrade, Serbia 2022.

Dzudovic, B., Dzudovic, J., Subotic, B., Obradovic, S. Antithrombin activity is a significant predictor of early mortality in pulmonary embolism patients. *Vojnosanitpregl.* (2021); Online First December, 2021.

Dzudovic, B., Subotic, B., Novicic, N., Matijasevic, J., Trobok, J., Miric, M., Salinger-Martinovic, S., Stanojevic, D., Nikolic, M., Miloradovic, V., Nikolic, N. M., Dekleva, M., Stefanovic, D.L., Kos Lj, Preradovic, T.K., Obradovic, S. Sex-related difference in the prognostic value of syncope for 30-day mortality among hospitalized pulmonary embolism patients. *Clin. Respir. J.* (2020) 14(7):645-651.

Dzudovic, J. Differences among the factors of coagulation cascade, and blood concentration of fibrinogen and D-dimer in patients with acute treated with direct oral anticoagulants. *Military Medical Academy, School of Medicine, University of Defense* 2022.

Dzudovic, J., Dzudovic, B., Subota, V., Antunovic, M., Stavri, M., Subotic, B., Obradovic, S. Differences between activities of coagulation factors after one month of therapy with different direct oral anticoagulant in pulmonary embolism patients. *J. Clin. Pharm. Ther.* (2019) 44(2):236-242.

Dzudovic, J., Crevar Sakac, M., Antunovic, M., Repic, A., Obradovic, S., Djordjevic, S., Savic, J., Djudovic, B. Development and validation of LC-MS/MS method for determination of plasma apixaban. *Acta Chromatographica* (2022) 34:332–337.

Goldhaber, S. Z., Visani, L., De Rosa, M. Acute pulmonary embolism: clinical outcomes in the International Cooperative Pulmonary Embolism Registry (ICOPER). *Lancet* (1999) 353(9162)1386-1389.

Jovanović, L j. Value of biomarkers measurements form the blood to acute pulmonary embolism outcome in respect of the ethology. *Doctor thesis, Scholl of Medicine Kragujevac, University of Kragujevac* 2021.

Jovanovic, Lj., Rajkovic, M., Subota, V., Subotic, B., Dzudovic, B., Matijasevic, J., Benic, M., Salinger, S., Simovic, S., Miloradovic, V., Kovacevic, T. P., Kos, Lj., Neskovic, A., Kafedzic, S., Nikolic, N. M., Bozovic, B., Bulatovic, N., Obradovic, S. Predictive value of admission glycemia in diabetics with pulmonary embolism compared to non-diabetic patients· *Acta Diabetologica* (2022); 59(5):653-659.

Jovanović, Lj., Subota, V., Stavrić, M., Dzudovic, B., Subotic, B.,Novic, N., Miric, M., Matijasevic, J., Nikolic, M., Miloradovic, V., Salinger, S., Nikolic, N. M., Kos,Lj., Preradovic, T.K, Obradovic, S. Different predictive value for short-term all-cause mortality with commonly used biomarkers regarding the cause of pulmonary embolism. *Vojnosanit Pregl.* (2021) 78(5):542–548.

Jovanovic, Lj., Subota, V., Stavric, M., Subotic, B., Dzudovic, B., Novicic, N., Matijasevic, J., Miric, M., Salinger, S., Nikolic, N. M., Nikolic, M., Miloradovic, V., Kos,Lj., Preradovic, T. K., Marinkovic, J., Kocev, N., Obradovic, S. Biomarkers for the prediction of early pulmonary embolism related mortality in spontaneous and provoked thrombotic disease. *Clin. Chim. Acta* (2019) 492:78-83.

Matijašević, J., Mirić, M., Trobok-Vučićević, J., Andrijevic, I., Dzudovic, B., Subotic, B., Obradovic, S.Sex-specific differences and risk factors for 30-day mortality in acute pulmonary embolism – Results from the Serbian Multicenter Pulmonary Embolism Registry. *Vojnosanitpregl.* (2021) 78(12):1263-1272.

Meyer, G., Vicaut, E., Danays, T., Agnelli, G., Becattini, C., Beyer-Westendorf, J., Bluhmki, E., Bouvaist, H., Brenner, B., Couturaud, F., Dellas, C., Empen, K., Franca, A., Galiè, N., Geibel, A., Goldhaber, S. Z., Jimenez, D, Kozak, M., Kupatt, K., Kucher, N., Lang, I. M., Lankeit, M., Meneveau, N., Pacouret, G., Palazzini, M., Petris, A., Pruszczyk, P., Rugolotto, M., Salvi, A., Schellong, S., Sebbane, M., Sobkowicz, B., Stefanovic, B. S., Thiele, H., Torbicki, A., Verschuren, F., Konstantinides, S. V.; PEITHO Investigators. Fibrinolysis for patients with intermediate-risk pulmonary embolism. *N Engl J Med* (2014) 370:1402–11.

Milić, R. Value of C-reactive protein in serum in patients with acute pulmonary embolism. *Doctor thesis, School of Medicine* Kragujevac, University of Kragujevac 2018.

Milić, R., Džudović, B., Subotić, B., Obradovic, S., Soldatovic, I., Petrovic, M. The significance of C-reactive protein for the prediction of net-adverse clinical outcome in patients with acute pulmonary embolism. *Vojnosanit. Pregl.* (2019) 76 (4): 431–436.

Monreal, M., Jiménez, D., Bikdeli, B. RIETE Registry: Past, Present and Future. *Arch. Bronconeumol.* (2022) 58(3):205-207.

Novicic, N., Dzudovic, B., Subotic, B., Salinger-Martimovic, S., Obradovic, S. Electrocardiography changes and their significance during treatment of patients with intermediate-high and high-risk pulmonary embolism. *Eur. Heart J. Acute Cardiovasc. Care.* (2019) 9(4):271-278.

Obradovic, S., Dzudovic, B., Subotic, B., Matijasevic, J., Mladenovic, Z., Bokan, A., Trobok, J., Pekovic, S., Salinger-Martinovic, S., Jovanovic,Lj., Kos,Lj., Kovacevic-Preradovic, T., Nikolic, M., Miloradovic, V., Kovacevic-Kuzmanovic, A., Zec, N., Markovic-Nikolic, N.,Srdanovic, I., Gluvic, Z., Kafedzic, S., Pancevacki, S., Neskovic, A. and Konstantinides, S. Predictive value of heart failure with reduced versus preserved ejection fraction for outcome in pulmonary embolism. *ESC Heart Failure* (2020) 7(6):4061-4070.

Obradović, S., Rusović, S., Gligić. B. *Pulmonary embolism through the case reports. Monography, Belgrade* 2011.

Obradovic, S., Subotic, B., Dzudovic, B., Matijasevic, J., Dzudovic, J/, Salinger-Martinovic, S., Miloradovic, V., Preradovic, T. K., Marinkovic, J., Neskovic, A. Pulmonary embolism bleeding score index (PEBSI): A new tool for the detection of patients with low risk for major bleeding on thrombolytic therapy. *Thromb Res* (2022) 214:138-143.

Obradovic, S. D., Dzudovic, B. M., Subotic, B. N., Dzudovic, J. M., Matijasevic, J. A., Benic, M. D., Trobok, J. L., Pekovic, S.M., Salinger-Martinovic, S., Jovanovic, Lj., Kos, Lj., Preradovic, T.K., Simovic, S.M., Miloradovic, V.M., Kuzmanovic, A. M., Mrdjan, T. D., Bozovic, B. Z., Bulatovic, N. S., Kafedzic, S.V., Pancevacki, S., Neskovic, A.N. Prognostic significance of symptomatic deep vein thrombosis in patients with acute symptomatic pulmonary embolism regarding the European Society of Cardiology mortality risk model. *Int. Angiol.* (2022) 41(4):338-5.

Pruszczyk, P., Klok, F. A., Kucher, N., Roik, M., Meneveau, N., Sharp, A.S., Nielsen-Kudsk, J. E., Obradović, S., Barco, S., Giannini, S., Stefanini, G, Tarantini, G., Konstantinides S, Dudek D. Percutaneous treatment options for acute pulmonary embolism: a clinical consensus statement by the ESC Working Group on pulmonary circulation and right ventricular function and the European Association of Percutaneous Cardiovascular Interventions. *Eurointervention* (2022)18(8): e623-e38.

Ruzicic, D., Dzudovic, B., Matijasevic, J., Salinger, S., Kos,Lj., Preradovic, T. K., Mitevska, I., Neskovic, A., Bozovic, B.,Bulatovic, N., Miloradovic, V.. Djuric, I, and Obradovic, O. Signs and symptoms of acute pulmonary embolism and their predictive value for all-cause hospital death in respect of severity of the disease, age, sex, and body mass index: retrospective analysis of the Regional PE Registry (REPER). *BMJ OA Resp Res* (2023) in press.

Salinger-Martinovic, S., Dimitrijevic, Z., Stanojevic, D., Momčilović, S., Kostic, T., Koracevic, G., Subotic, B., Dzudovic, B., Stefanovic, B.,Matijasevic, J.,Miric, M., Nikolic, N. M., Nikolic, M., Miloradovic, V., Kos,Lj., Preradovic, T.K., Srdanovic, I., Stanojevic, J.,Obradovic, O. Renal dysfunction as intrahospital prognostic indicator in acute pulmonary embolism. *Int. J. Cardiol.* (2020) 302:143-149.

Schulman, S., Kearon C.; Definition of major bleeding in clinical investigations of antihemostatic medicinal products in non-surgical patients. *J. Thromb. Haemost.* 2005 Apr;3(4):692-4.

Sekulić, I. Comparative analysis of four therapeutic protocols in patients with intermediate-high risk acute pulmonary embolism. *Doctor Thesis, School of Medicine Kragujevac, University of Kragujevac* 2019.

Sekulic, I., Dzudovic, B., Matijasevic, J., Batranovic, U., Rusovic, S., Mihajlovic, M., Miladinovic, U., Rancic, N., Subotic, B., Novicic, N., Gavrilovic, S., Sekulic, J.B., Obradovic, S. Ultrasound assisted thrombolysis in intermediate-risk patients with pulmonary thromboembolism. *Acta Cardiol.* (2019) 75(7):623-630.

Tritschler T., Kraaijpoel N., Philippe Girard P., Büller H. P., Langlois, N., Righini, M., Schulman, S., Segers, A., Le Gal, G.; Subcommittee on Predictive and Diagnostic Variables in Thrombotic Disease. Definition of pulmonary embolism-related death and classification of the cause of death in venous thromboembolism studies: Communication from the SSC of the ISTH. *J. Thromb Haemost.* 2020 Jun;18(6):1495-1500.

Yamashita, Y., Morimoto, T., Amano, H, Takase, T., Hiramori, S., Kim, K., Oi, M., Akao, M., Kobayashi, Y., Toyofuku, M., Izumi, T.,Tada, T.,Chen, P., Murata, K., Tsuyuki, Y., Saga, S., Sasa, T., Sakamoto, J., Kinoshita, M., Togi, K., Mabuchi, H., Takabayashi, K., Shiomi, H., Kato, T., Makiyama T., Ono, K., Takeshi Kimura, T. Validation of simplified PESI score for identification of low-risk patients with pulmonary embolism: From the COMMAND VTE Registry. *Eur. Heart J. Acute Cardiovasc. Care.* 2020 Jun; 9(4):262-270.

Zhang, S., Xu, X., Ji, Y., Takase, T., Hiramori, S., Kim, K., Oi, M., Akao, M., Kobayashi, Y., Toyofuku, M., Izumi, T., Tada, T., Chen, P.M., Murata, K., Tsuyuki, Y., Saga, S., Sasa, T., Sakamoto, J., Kinoshita, M., Togi, K., Mabuchi, H.,Takabayashi, K., Shiomi, H., Kato, T., Makiyama, T., Ono, K., Kimura, T. Clinical phenotypes with prognostic implications in pulmonary embolism patients with syncope. CURES Registry. *Front Cardiovasc. Med.* (2022) 9:836850.

Chapter 13

Pulmonary Embolism Response Team (PERT): A Multidisciplinary Approach to Pulmonary Embolism Treatment

Slobodan Obradovic*, PhD
Clinic of Cardiology, Military Medical Academy,
School of Medicine University of Defense, Belgrade, Serbia

Abstract

The treatment approach for patients with intermediate and high-risk pulmonary embolism (PE) is a challenging area with continuing controversial opinions and ongoing scientific research. There is a major evolution of medical and invasive therapeutic approaches, although fast and practical treatment decisions in emergency settings can often be difficult. Complex cases necessitate the involvement of multiple specialties in the care of patients with acute PE. The aim of creating pulmonary embolism response teams (PERTs) is to improve the organization of care and response to serious PE patients. Those teams are organized by many hospitals and academic clinical centers world widely. The main goal of the PERT is to organize a multidisciplinary team of experts in thromboembolic disease, who can give a fast response in patients with acute PE, offer consultations, and provide practical use of the wide therapeutic options in the acute treatment phase. There is much scientific data that have confirmed the value of PERTs in the improvement of patient outcomes, and reduction of hospitalization and health care costs.

* Corresponding Author's Email: sloba.d.obradovic@gmail.com.

In: Pulmonary Embolism
Editors: Irena Mitevska, Sonja Salinger, Marijan Bosevski et al.
ISBN: 979-8-89113-175-0

Keywords: advanced therapies, multidisciplinary teams, pulmonary embolism

Introduction

Pulmonary embolism (PE) is one of the world's leading causes of morbidity and mortality and one of the most missed diagnoses. Heterogenous clinical presentations ranging from asymptomatic, mild forms to hemodynamic instability with obstructive shock, make diagnosis challenging. Over the past decades, many clinical trials and guidelines established diagnostic pathways based on PE probability assessment, medical, interventional and surgical treatment options for individual PE patients. However, despite all these developments mortality in high-risk PE patients still remains high (Kucher et al., 2006, Secemsky et al., 2018). Treatment doubts that appear in more complex cases, often based on variable experts' opinion and treatment decisions, lead to formation of multidisciplinary pulmonary embolism response team (PERT) focused on PE treatment across the world.

Pulmonary Embolism Response Team: Aim and Activities

The pulmonary embolism response team (PERT) is a multidisciplinary medical team which deals with complex pulmonary embolism management. The problem of management of acute PE is that PE is a complication of many diseases and conditions rather than being a certain entity per se. In such a way, acute pulmonary embolism should be treated with various specialists and their combined knowledge is really needed for the proper treatment. On the other hand, no single specialist has all the necessary knowledge and skills for the individual PE patient. One of the consequences of this is that the guidelines on the PE management are full of serious gaps and even contradictions in the situation where we have not enough evidence-based data on many issues. For instance, the European Society of Cardiology (ESC) 2019 guidelines do not recommend thrombolytic therapy in patients with intermediate-high acute PE, mostly according to one big randomized trial (Meyer et al., 2014) which used only one thrombolytic protocol with tenecteplasis, where even this trial demonstrated that this therapy significantly decreases the primary end point, the composite of death and hemodynamic decompensation within 7 days after randomization since the rate of major bleeding (but not fatal bleeding) was too high. Many physicians who deal with PE consider that reperfusion therapy is needed in much wider indications than guidelines (Konstantinides et al., 2019), and evidence-based medicine is recommended, but we do not know which is the best reperfusion therapy for various subgroups of patients. Catheter-directed therapy is a valuable option, but it needs trained staff with the various possibilities of this option, from aspiration to mechanical or thrombolytic thrombus fragmentation. The decision to use reperfusion therapy or not is the crucial question during the management of PE patients (Kabrhel et al., 2016; Barnes et al., 1995). Continuous estimation of PE-related death risk and bleeding risk is necessary for the proper decision. The current guidelines are somehow conservative and do not allow the preventive use of reperfusion therapy before hemodynamic collapse when the risk of dying becomes too high. The decision to use reperfusion is often very complex, because the estimation of bleeding risk and the option for reperfusion sometime need the expertise of various specialties. Also, the use of extracorporeal membrane oxygenation (ECMO) therapy needs a high degree of expertise and also needs decisions of several specialties (Hobohm et al., 2022).

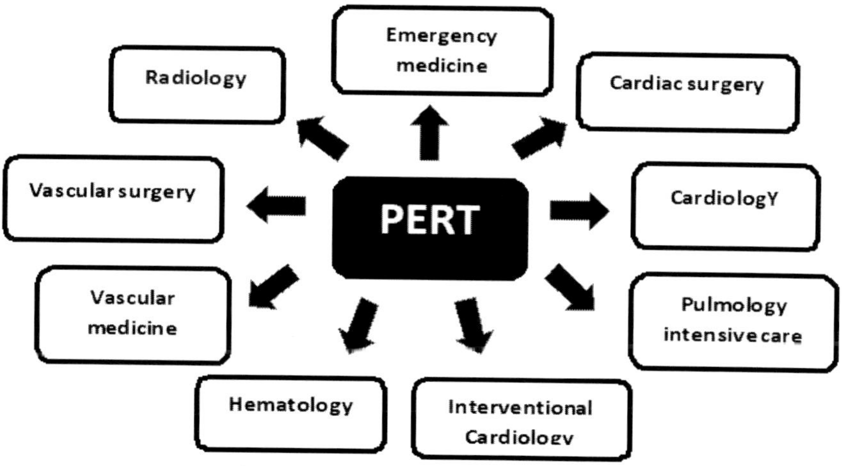

Abbreviations: PERT- pulmonary embolism response team.

Figure 1. Example of the main PERT participating specialists.

All this is imposed from the institutions who manage PE patients to develop multidisciplinary teams to use all available resources to overcome various obstacles in the treatment of PE patients which are more the rule than the exception (Barnes et al., 2016, Rosovsky et al., 2018). The composition of the Pulmonary Embolism Response teams is different in different institutions and depends on the local expertise and equipment (Corrigan et al., 2016). Generally, intensivists, interventional cardiologists, radiologists, cardio-surgeons, and pulmonologists are the core of such teams and many other specialists could be engaged if it is necessary. An example shown in Figure 1.

The main aim of the PERT is the prompt evaluation of complex patients and to take responsibility for the treatment option they choose for specific patients. Many possible clinical problems could be the tasks for the PERT team (Table 1). The leader of the team must be closely related to the patient, experienced, and have a team spirit which enables engagement of the necessary and right resources for the best management of the particular patient. He or she also must have the authority and power to organize various diagnostic and therapeutic procedures (Dudzinski DM et al., 2017, Galmer et al., 2017, Huisman et al., 2017).

Written protocols considering various anticipated clinical problems should be established with continuous improvement of PE management.

Table 1. Clinical problems which are the main goals for the PERT

Clinical problem	Specialty
Estimation of patient's risk of dying from PE	Radiology, echocardiography, laboratory, intensivist
Choice of appropriate reperfusion therapy.	Interventional radiology or cardiology, cardiac or vascular surgeon
Estimation of patient's risk for bleeding and treatment of bleeding	Transfusiology, hematology, surgeon, gastrointestinal endoscopy specialist, intensivist
Use of ECMO	Intensivist, vascular surgeons
Intensive respiratory support	Intensivist, pulmonology, cardiology
Early discharge	Various specialties
Treatment of oncology patients	Oncologist, clinical pharmacology, various specialty in respect of the kind, stage and location of malignant disease
Treatment of pregnant patients	Gynecology, anesthesiology, transfusiology
Communication with the PE network	Consultancy, organization of transport of more complex patients who could not be adequately treated in some hospitals, education of the network members

Abbreviations: ECMO- extracorporeal membrane oxygenation.

It is also important to develop an external network with other institutions to help them with advice or with the possibility to transfer patients to those facilities which give the patient the best chance to cure.

Many investigations have shown that the use of PERT means advanced patient care in acute PE, and PERT is the recommended way of treatment by the ESC 2019 PE guidelines (Konstantinides et al., 2019).

The large, recently published meta-analysis of 16 studies and more than 3,000 PERT-treated patients compared to a similar size control group concluded that PERT patients had a greater chance of being treated with catheter-directed therapy, venous-arterial (V-A) ECMO, surgical embolectomy, and all these procedures significantly decrease mortality compared to controls (Sosa et al., 2022).

Conclusion

Pulmonary embolism response teams are necessary for the management of acute PE patients in large, multidisciplinary hospitals because the complexity of the acute PE patients can require different kinds of expertise for adequate, personalized PE treatment.

References

Barnes, G., Giri, J., Courtney, D. M., Naydenov, S., Wood, T., Rosovsky, R., Rosenfield, K., Kabrhel, C.; National PERT™ Consortium Research Committee. Nuts and bolts of running a pulmonary embolism response team: results from an organizational survey of the National PERT Consortium members. *Hosp. Pract.* 1995; 45:76–80.

Barnes, G. D., Kabrhel, C., Courtney, D. M., Naydenov, S., Wood, T., Rosovsky, R., Rosenfield, K., Giri, J.; National PERT Consortium Research Committee. Diversity in the pulmonary embolism response team model: an organizational Survey of the National PERT Consortium members. *Chest.* 2016; 150:1414–7.

Corrigan, D., Prucnal, C., Kabrhel, C. Pulmonary embolism: the diagnosis, risk-stratification, treatment and disposition of emergency department patients. *Clin. Exp. Emerg. Med.* 2016; 3:117–25.

Dudzinski, D. M., Giri, J., Rosenfield, K. Interventional treatment of pulmonary embolism. *Circ. Cardiovasc. Interv.* 2017; 10:pii:e004345.

Galmer, A., Weinberg, I., Giri, J., Jaff, M., Weinberg, M. The role of the pulmonary embolism response team: how to build one, who to include, scenarios, organization, and algorithms. *Tech. Vasc. Interv. Radiol.* 2017; 20:216–23.

Hobohm, L., Sagoschen, I., Habertheuer, A., Barco, B., Valerio, L., Wild, J., Schmidt, F. P., Gori, T., Münzel, T., Konstantinides, S., Keller, K. Clinical use and outcome of extracorporeal membrane oxygenation in patients with pulmonary embolism. *Resuscitation* (2022) 170 285-292.

Huisman, M. V., Montero, Cabezas, J. M., Klok, F. A. Pulmonary embolism response teams: what is the added value for patients with acute pulmonary embolism? *Ned. TijdschrGeneeskd.* 2017;161: D1570.

Kabrhel, C., Rosovsky, R., Channick, R., Jaff, M. R., Weinberg, I., Sundt, T., Dudzinski, D. M., Rodriguez-Lopez, J. R., Parry, B. A., Harshbarger, S., Chang, Y., Rosenfield, K. A multidisciplinary pulmonary embolism response team: initial 30-month experience with a novel approach to delivery of care to patients with submassive and massive pulmonary embolism. *Chest.* 2016; 150:384–93.

Konstantinides, S. V., Meyer, G., Becattini, C., Bueno, H., Geersing, G. J., Harjola, V. P., Huisman, M. V., Humbert, M., Jennings, C. S., Jiménez, D., Kucher, N., Lang, I. M., Lankeit, M., Lorusso, R., Mazzolai, L., Meneveau, N., Áinle, F. N., Prandoni, P., Pruszczyk, P., Righini, M., Torbicki, A., Belle, E. V., Zamorano, J. L.; ESC Scientific Document Group. ESC Guidelines for the diagnosis and management of acute pulmonary embolism developed in collaboration with the European Respiratory Society (ERS). *Eur. Heart J.* 2020 Jan 21;41(4):543-603.

Kucher, N., Rossi, E., De Rosa, M., Goldhaber, S. Z. Massive pulmonary embolism. *Circulation*. 2006; 113:577–82.

Meyer, G., Vicaut, E., Danays, T., Agnelli, G., Becattini, C., Beyer-Westendorf, J., Bluhmki, E., Bouvaist, H., Brenner, B., Couturaud, F., Dellas, C., Empen, K., Franca, A., Galiè, N., Geibel, A., Goldhaber, S. Z., Jimenez, D., Kozak, M., Kupatt, K., Kucher, N., Lang, I. M., Lankeit, M., Meneveau, N., Pacouret, G., Palazzini, M.. Petris, A., Pruszczyk, P., Rugolotto, M., Salvi, A., Schellong, S., Sebbane, M., Sobkowicz, B., Stefanovic, B. S., Thiele, H., Torbicki, A, Verschuren, F., Konstantinides, S. V.; PEITHO Investigators. Fibrinolysis for patients with intermediate-risk pulmonary embolism. *N. Engl. J. Med.* (2014) 370:1402–11.

Rosovsky, R., Borges, J., Kabrhel, C., Rosenfield, K. Pulmonary embolism response team: inpatient structure, outpatient follow-up, and is it the current standard of care? *Clin. Chest Med.* 2018; 39:621–30.

Secemsky, E., Chang, Y., Jain, C. C., Beckman, J. A., Giri, J., Jaff, M. R., Rosenfield, K., Rosovsky, R., Kabrhel, C., Weinberg, I. Contemporary management and outcomes of patients with massive and submassive pulmonary embolism. *Am. J. Med.* 2018; 131:1506–14.

Sosa, D. F., Lehr, A. L., Zhao, H., Roth, S., Lakhther, V., Bashir, R., Cohen, G., Panaro, J., Maldonado, T. S., Horowitz, J., Amoroso, N. E., Criner, G. J., Shari, B., Brosnahan, S. B., Rali, P. Impact of pulmonary embolism response teams on acute pulmonary embolism: a systematic review and meta-analysis. *Eur. Respir. Rev.* (2022) 31 220023.

About the Editors

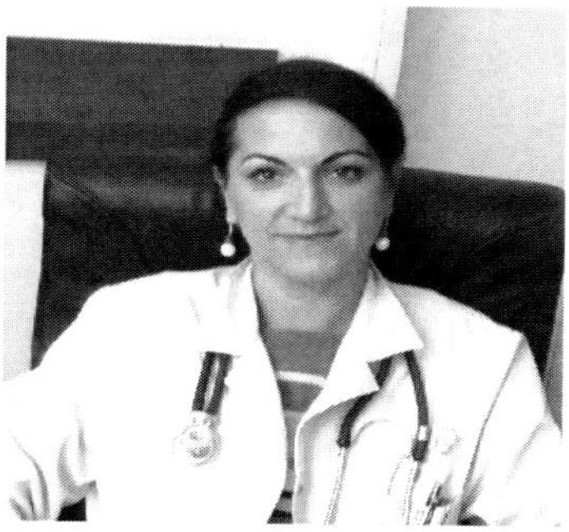

Irena Mitevska
University Cardiology Clinic, Medical Faculty University
"St. Cyril and Metodij" Skopje, North Macedonia

Associate Prof. Dr. Irena Mitevska received her PhD from Medical Faculty, University "St. Cyril and Methodius" in Skopje, North Macedonia in 2017. Now, she is working as an Associate Professor at the University Cardiology Clinic, Medical Faculty in Skopje, North Macedonia. She is a part of Intensive care Unit, echocardiography and nuclear imaging consultant. Dr Mitevska is a Vice President of the National Society of Cardiology of North Macedonia and an active member of several international cardiology societies. Associate Prof. Mitevska is committed to the research, diagnosis and treatment of acute cardiac pathology including pulmonary embolism, heart failure and coronary artery disease. So far, she has published more than 60 scientific papers as the first author of coauthor in national and international cardiology journals. She has been involved and is actively working in several multicentric randomized trials and registries, such as SIGNIFY Trial, ISCHEMIA trial, HERMES Trials, REPER Pulmonary Embolism regional registry, as well as several registries of the European Society of Cardiology, including registry on Heart

Failure III and Non-STEMI registry. She has been Co-author of two chapters in the book published by NOVA Science Publishers: "Cardio diabetes".

E-mail: peovskai@yahoo.com

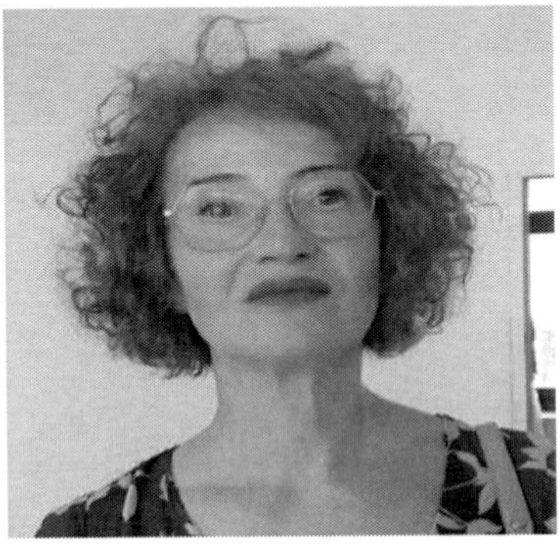

Sonja Salinger
Cardiology Clinic, Medical Faculty, University of NIs
Nis, Sebia

Associate Professor Dr. Sonja Slinger received her PhD from Medical Faculty, University "of Nis in 2001. Now, she is working as an Associate professor at the Cardiology Clinic, University of Nis in Serbia. Dr Salinger is Consultant in Interventional Cardiology, Oncology and Echocardiography. She is a member of the Women Committee of the European Society of Cardiology (ESC) PCI (EAPCI) as well as ESC Council of Cardio oncology. Dr Salinger is an interventional Cardiologist, educated in several clinical cardiology centers including Institute of Dedinje in Serbia and Kerckhof Klinik Bad Nauheim in Germany. Associate professor Salinger participated in international studies including Multicentric CENTURY Study.

Dr Salinger is actively involved in diagnosis and treatment of acute cardiovascular disease including pulmonary embolism, heart failure and acute coronary syndromes. So far, she has published more than 100 scientific papers as the first author of coauthor in national and international cardiology journals. She is an active member of the regional registry on pulmonary embolism REPER.

E-mail: sonja.salinger@gmail.com

Index

D

E

G

H

I

W